Transformation: Treating Trauma with Acupuncture and Herbs is perhaps the most important book yet written on the subject of trauma in the field of acupuncture and Oriental medicine. Dr. Morris makes a major contribution to trauma treatment with his pioneering techniques. Expect to see radical improvements in your patients when using Dr. Morris' treatment protocol. This is a powerful medicine. Dr. Morris' book is a must-read for every acupuncturist who treats trauma.

Constance "Ahuva Batya" Scharff, PhD
Director of Addiction Research, Cliffside Malibu
Author and Speaker

In *Transformation: Treating Trauma with Acupuncture and Herbs*, Dr. William Morris thoughtfully weaves ecological, psychological, and social concepts with that of classical Chinese. The foundations derive from Dr. Morris' tireless examination of classical Chinese literature, fascination with psychology, and more than thirty-six years of clinical experience. While some practitioners disregard secondary vessels as antiquated, Dr. Morris masterfully brings them alive in an original and clinically relevant way.

Joseph Adams, LAc

This work has transformed my own path of healing as well as that of each of my patients. After studying and putting this approach into practice, I can say unequivocally that it will dramatically increase the positive progression of healing traumatic wounds, both emotional and physical.

Jon Dollar, LAc

The profection method for treating current manifestations of past trauma is extraordinary. Not only does it help to relieve current symptoms, but it also works to release the original pattern of trauma. Combining profection with extraordinary vessel treatment strategies, I have witnessed profound clinical transformations in numerous patients.

Thomas Richardson, LAc, MTS

TRANSFORMATION

TREATING TRAUMA
WITH
ACUPUNCTURE AND HERBS

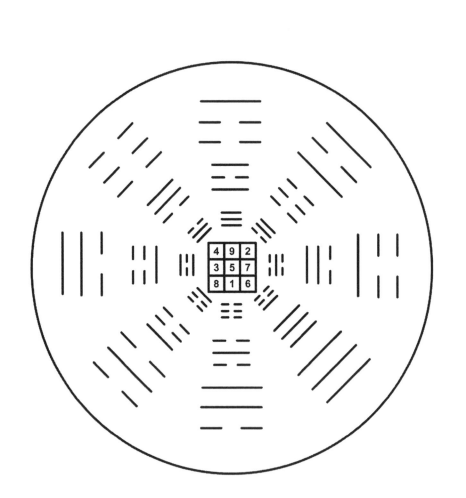

TRANSFORMATION

TREATING TRAUMA
WITH
ACUPUNCTURE AND HERBS

WILLIAM MORRIS, PH.D.

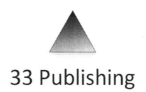

33 Publishing

TRANSFORMATION
TREATING TRAUMA WITH ACUPUNCTURE AND HERBS

Copyright © 2015 William Morris

ISBN: 978-1-941142-85-1

TABLE OF CONTENTS

TABLE OF FIGURES

TABLE OF TABLES

ACKNOWLEDGEMENTS

First, respect and gratitude go to those historic characters whose contributions make a work such as this possible. Bian Que, and Wang Shu-he provide a foundation for the Chinese medical theory. Wilhelm Reich, Stanislov Grof, and Jean Piaget provided a platform for the development of important philosophical features of this work. Respect, also to my teachers John H.F. Shen and Leon Hammer who provided a foundation of thought that made a work such as this possible.

This book is dedicated to students of the art of pulse diagnosis in clinical practice. There are those who participate in the direct lineage, keeping this work alive. Special thanks to the individuals who have assisted in the teaching of this material: Joe Adams, Jay Bulloch, Jon Dollar, Mary Nicosia, Tom Richardson, and Pam Fischer. Also, those people who keep the material alive in their practices, in preparation to teach: Kelsey Barrett, Jay Sol Bartlett, Madelaina Bolduc, Ben Broadhead, Ellen Evans, Krista Raven Herbe, Christina Korpik, Ann Mowat, Jonny Nobleza, Katie Novotny, Tony Siefert. Constance Scharff served as sounding board and editor. Finally, I want to thank Allan Combs; my studies with him became the inspiration for this book.

Special thanks, also, to my mother and father who brought me here and gave me the tools that appear throughout this work. Great appreciation goes to my children, Joshua, Solena, and Zoe. Thank you, also, to Bobbie Morris who supported me during the early stages of this work. Appreciation is given to Colleen Morris, who supported me during the middle efforts. Lastly, I send love and appreciation to Mary Nicosia who is actively involved in supporting this work.

FOREWORD

Any sufficiently advanced technology is indistinguishable from magic.
—Sir Arthur C. Clarke's Third Law[1]

In this remarkable little book, Dr. Morris lays out the basics for a form of medical assessment, as well as a form of treatment that may seem strange to the Western reader, perhaps even uncanny or magical. Many readers will, for the first time, find themselves before a radically different conception of the human organism, one that is profoundly holistic and based on an entirely different history of thought and practice than that to which they are accustomed. It may, at first, seem primitive or completely non-rational. Nevertheless, it represents the result of its own long and evolving tradition of medical observation and practice.

The interested reader will especially appreciate Dr. Morris' descriptions of physical and psychological growth and transformation. In the following pages, he gives us a unique understanding of how the mind and body gather themselves into distinct changes of state. He not only clarifies the deep meaning of change and transformation in Chinese thought, but substantially contributes to Western psychological knowledge as well. Here we are given a remarkable collection of ideas from the present and from the past, even the ancient past, all conspiring to enrich our understanding of human growth and transformation in all ways and on all levels.

It may seem strange to think of the Chinese civilization as offering an advanced technology, but it is well to recall that it is one

---

[1] Clarke, Arthur C. (1984/1962). *Profiles of the Future: An Inquiry Into the Limits of the Possible.* New York: Holt, Rinehart & Wilson. pp. 205n. ISBN 0030697832.

of the oldest civilizations on earth, and through time has developed its own philosophies and technologies almost independently of the influence of the West. These ideas have also exerted considerable influence on Japanese culture and reflect a worldview dramatically different than that which dominates in the West. In contrast, the philosophies of India tend to have a natural simpatico with the Western Abrahamic worldviews of Christianity, Judaism, and Islam. All of the latter hold the ideal of a single overarching deity or principle, whether in the form of Brahman or Jehovah. It is, perhaps, for this reason that European culture so easily embraced the philosophies of India in a friendly manner not long after the Enlightenment, while Chinese nontheistic philosophies such as Confucianism, Buddhism, Taoism, and Taoist-influenced forms of Buddhism, such as Chen in China and Zen in Japan, have taken serious root in the West only during the second half of the 20th century.

Taoism is especially important to our present story because it presents a radically holistic and organic view of all aspects of life. The *Tao* is a name for the fundamental process of growth and change that undergirds and embraces the entire manifest universe. According to Taoism, all life is rooted in the flowing, living essence of the Tao. This way of thinking is poles apart from traditional Western deistic notions of the existence of a Creator beyond the physical world, or the Enlightenment conception of Newton's clockwork universe, governed mathematically by physical "laws."[2] It gives birth to an entirely different view of health in the human body and mind, one that includes implicit notions of growth and transformation imbued in the very fabric of human life as well as the cosmos in general. This in mind, it is not surprising that Chinese thinking about physical and mental health allow for transformations through successive stages of maturation.

---

[2] A notion that can be traced back historical to the Christian idea of the "laws of God," imparted on the manifest cosmos in the act of creation itself.

At the same time, the fundamental Buddhist notion of *dependent origination*, widely understood historically in China, emphasizes a systemic view of the human condition. It is a vision of the integrity of nature and the human being as networked interlocking systems, symbolized by the image of Indra's Net,[3] in which all aspects of the cosmos are seen like gems, each reflecting back images of all the others. It is also represented as mirrors, each one reflecting images of the others in a single unified network. In Chinese thought, the notion of co-arising, always and everywhere undergirded by the *Tao*, provides a vision of the human condition, both psychologically and organically, as growing and changing, embedded in an ever-arising web of interconnected physical and social conditions.

Needless to say, Western notions of medicine typically derive from scientific investigations of disease. Like most, if not all, of Western science since the Enlightenment, these have tended to emphasize single causal agents and the unique symptoms they elicit. Medical understanding of the human body and mind has only, in recent decades, begun to take into account a broader spectrum of influences that act upon an individual, giving rise to a total state of health or disease. Much has been written about this topic, but it is safe to say that few Western scientists, and even fewer physicians, have yet to acquire a deep appreciation of the importance of the whole human organism in its social and natural world as the basis for assessment of health and the establishment of treatment programs.

Allan Combs, Ph.D.
California Institute of Integral Studies
Author of *The Radiance of Being*, etc.

---

[3] An idea said to have originated in the Chinese Huayan school of Buddhism.

Introduction

This book is about the transformation of relationships, both internally between aspects of self and externally with others, ultimately transcending such dualisms. Combining Western psychiatric views on the protective systems of armoring with Chinese medicine, the works of Wilhelm Reich and Stanislov Grof, I weave a fabric of theory and practice.

Grounding self within the constitution, the traumatic impacts of life are explored and treatment strategies are developed. This work provides tools for interacting with and transforming the decisions that people use to create their lives. For, as an important mentor to me, Leon Hammer, said, "People do what they do in order to survive, even if it kills them."

Trauma scatters vitality. If it is sufficient to cause shock, it leaves an imprint which tends to be heightened during transitions between life stages. If, for example, a child experiences shock such as the divorce of parents, they often believe that they are the cause. This is, in part, due to the magical world-view of the child. As puberty develops, the emphasis is on defining self in the context of relationship. The life story created in response to a shock at this stage has a lasting impact on the individual and the possibilities of their relationships. Shocks in early adulthood lead to stories that are built around purpose for being, related to livelihood.

The ideas we create as a defense against the traumatic and painful parts of life eventually arrive in the body. As transformation and release takes place, it is important that it take place from upper regions of the body to the lower. Begin with the ocular region, the jaw, neck, chest, diaphragm, and eventually the pelvis. It is important not to create discharge and release from lower segments as the energy can rise, increasing the sense of blockage above (Reich, 1980a; 1980b).

The materials of this book are woven of practice, literature, and "mouth-to-ear and action-to-sight transmission" in a participatory clinical experience. Such knowledge is placed into a feedback system through classroom environs and publications. It is thus built from a constructivist and participatory world view, open to revision and critique.

The implications of this work are often deep and far-ranging. The practitioner is advised to ensure that the patient is in the care of a professional in the area of psychology when working through some of these materials.

Warmly,
William R. Morris, Ph.D.

THE SEVEN AGES OF MAN

All the world's a stage,
And all the men and women merely players:
They have their exits and their entrances;
And one man in his time plays many parts,
His acts being seven ages. At first the infant,
Mewling and puking in the nurse's arms.
Then the whining school-boy, with his satchel
And shining morning face, creeping like snail
Unwillingly to school. And then the lover,
Sighing like furnace, with a woeful ballad
Made to his mistress' eyebrow. Then a soldier,
Full of strange oaths, and bearded like the bard,
Jealous in honor, sudden and quick in quarrel,
Seeking the bubble reputation
Even in the cannon's mouth. And then the justice,
In fair round belly with good capon lined,
With eyes severe and beard of formal cut,
Full of wise saws and modern instances;
And so he plays his part. The sixth age shifts
Into the lean and slipper'd pantaloon,
With spectacles on nose and pouch on side,
His youthful hose, well saved, a world too wide
For his shrunk shank; and his big manly voice,
Turning again toward childish treble, pipes
And whistles in his sound. Last scene of all,
That ends this strange eventful history,
Is second childishness and mere oblivion,
Sans teeth, sans eyes, sans taste, sans everything.
—William Shakespeare

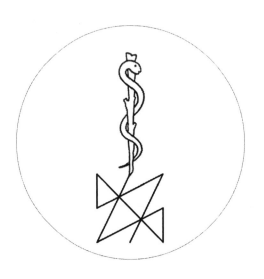

THE CONSTITUTIONAL SELF

Definition of Constitution

Individuals are rooted in the essence of the ancestors. This blood continuum from generation to generation heightens the importance of building treatments that take into consideration the family of Origen. From these hallowed halls, we evolve.

The idea of constitution provides a view into the essential nature of being. It refers to vitality, health, and strength in the physical. It can also be used to describe a person's mental or psychological makeup. One aspect of constitution can be built as the unique expression of that part of consciousness occurring as a thread of awareness of "I" over time. "Whereas space is central to the world of objects, time is central to the world of self" (Tulku 1984, p. 150).

Taxonomies are several by which we may organize this clinical gaze. Each medical culture has its approach and some have many. Ayurveda divides constitution into three forms of imbalance, fire (*pitta*), water (*kapha*) and air (*vata*). Fire relates to hot and quick-tempered people. Water people tend to hold fluid and move more slowly. The air person tends to be cold and changeable. The Greek system of Galen and Hippocrates uses a four-fold division of what are called humors: melancholic (cold and dry), choleric (hot and dry), sanguine (warm and moist), and phlegmatic (cold and moist).

Acupuncturists may use five transformations, pathogens, viscera and bowels or three treasures. Here is an example using the six external pathogens: wind, damp, cold, fire, summer heat, and heat. Windy people may be changeable and sensitive, damp people can hold fluids, cold people are often cold and retreating, while the fire person leans toward inflammatory conditions and a rather hot emotional temperament. The person with heat expresses more mildly than those with the more intense fire constitution. Summer heat people tend toward both dampness and heat, and can be vulnerable to the heat in the summer. One could also classify constitution according to the internal organs: a heart-type person, lungs, liver, kidneys, bladder, and so forth.

Famous 17th century English physician, Thomas Sydenham, viewed constitution as a complex set of natural events, including quality of soil, climate, seasons, rain, drought, and centers of pestilence, and famine. Rather than a fundamental nature, he suggests that constitution revolves around a hidden mystery. Such constitutions rarely have symptoms, nor are they defined by symptoms. The constitution is perceived in the relativity of differences—by a critical gaze (Sydenham 1979; Foucault 1963).

In the temporal frame, constitution may refer to the "I" presence, the bodily condition or the emotional tendency. It can be that continuity of being from the beginning of life. It also refers to acquired conditions over the course of life. And lastly, it can refer to stages of development (Jarrett 1999).

That aspect of constitution, which refers to the strength and integrity of the psychological and physical structures, has its roots in the kidneys according to Chinese medicine. Constitution, in terms of kidney essence, relates to innate strength and capacity of the individual, built like a tank or like a leaf blowing in the wind.

The Chinese medical concept of kidney includes the central nervous, skeletal, endocrine, reproductive, and urinary tract. These components of the kidney in Chinese medical thought provide platform for understanding the biopsychosocial capacities of the individual. The strength and adaptive capacity of these systems are part of the framework of constitution.

Spirit: Self Knowledge

First, we discuss the word *shen*, often translated as "spirit," and in this instance, a concept used both in the singular and plural. The singular aspect provides for the description of medical conditions such as disturbances of the psyche. The word "spirit" may further be used to describe an aggregate of conscious aspects of the self. The ideal spirit presents with a healthy, harmonious spiritedness. Spirit harmony and spiritedness include concepts such as unity, awareness, clarity, flexibility, stability, balance, power, reactivity, initiative, and processing (Yang and Morris, 2007).

Spirit resides within the heart, yet its five images find a resting place within the viscera. The incarnating and sensorial vitality of the *po* resides in the lungs. The transcendent dreamtime exponent of the *hun* lives in the liver. The creator mind of the *yi* projects all kinds of possibilities upon the world and lives in the spleen/pancreas. The will to action, called the *zhi*, resides in the kidneys. Yet, we can see in the works of the Indian saint Ramana Maharshi a focus upon a self-singular and transcendent to these facets of spirit in Chinese medicine. In this unity field of spirit, we find conscious being. The paradox between the singular and plural provides an access point for clinical interactions.

In the singular experience of self, the spirit travels the vessels residing in the heart. Spirit animates the singular physical body that operates as a commons for the collective intrapersonal selves. Externally, this becomes the ground upon which intersubjective experience is built.

The constitutional self, rooted in the kidneys and the essence discussed previously, provide a basis for the spirit. The kidneys also provide a home for the component of spirit called the will (*zhi*). *Zhi* brings forward both a *yin* will and a *yang* will. Carl Roger's notions of acceptance and undistorted experience of being, in order to become a complete and fully functioning organism, has similarity to a *yin* form of will (Rogers 1961). The ancient Chinese considered this to be accepting the will of heaven. The *yang* will involves those aspirations beyond the acceptance and undistorted experience of what is—the *yin*. Further, the *yang* will has that feature of intentionality which would overcome the seeming obstacles of life that the *yin* will would accept. The expansive nature aspires to liberation and a transcended state, while the *yin* contracting state engages in life, form, and the world.

This *shen* in the singular form presents with luminous clarity, sparkling like the stars in the sky. This *shen* consciousness is a superlogical state, contrasting to prelogical and logical states. Similar to the preconventional and conventional moral stages, prelogical rests closer to the ideations of early childhood, while the logic emerges in later childhood as a reasonable construction of the world.

The loss of spirit presents with dullness and flat affect. Chinese medical theory describes it as "spirit disturbance," which includes mental and spiritual pathological conditions. The patient's spiritedness may be evaluated by using the four examination methods of Chinese medical diagnosis: observation, olfaction, inquiry, and palpation.

Five Transformations

While controversial, I have found the methods of J.R. Worsley (1923–2003) to be of clinical use for identifying what he calls the *causative factor*. Such a label implies philosophical problems of causality, which are beyond the scope of this book. Therefore, I use the method for the purpose of identifying the constitution based upon the five elements (Worsley, 1990). The sound of the voice, the color of the temporal region, the emotions, and the odor of the individual are used to arrive at a sense of the constitution. Unschuld (1986) describes these correlations as a "doctrine of correspondences," whereby the associated features define, in this instance, a pattern of being.

The agents are identified via the sound, whether a shout (wood), laugh (fire), groan (water), sing-song (earth), or breathiness (metal). The facial colors around the temples are correspondingly: green, red, black, yellow, or white. And similarly for the emotions: anger, excess joy, fear, sympathy, and grief (please see Table 1).

It is through these more ephemeral qualities of expression in terms of feelings, sounds, and subtle facial colors that the essential components of self are determined. I use a further assessment of the life's purpose in order to grasp more firmly the constitutional nature of the individual.

Agent	Color	Sound	Emotion	Purpose
Fire	Red	Laughter	Joy	Connects
Earth	Yellow	Sing-song	Sympathy	Cares for
Metal	White	Breathiness	Grief	Stands for
Water	Bluish-Black	Deep groan	Fear	Seeks meaning
Wood	Greenish-Blue	Sharp and shouting	Anger	

Table 1: Five Transformations and Correspondences

Identity of the constitution (original self) can be discovered by asking a person about the past: where they grew up, and the nature of their relations. This form of inquiry allows the subject to become decompensated, thereby bringing forward a more authentic expression of the constitution (Jarrett, 1999). The expressions of constitution unfettered by noise of the present moment emerge and become apparent. Sounds, colors, and moods can all become more authentic to the root of being when uncoupled from the present. Parsing out the thematic emphasis of the person's life also helps to refine the constitutional assessment.

It is common for two constitutions to express during the interview. Seek out the dominant features. The second most dominant feature may be called a sub-type, whereby the individual expresses certain color, odor, sounds, emotions, and mission in a less dominant fashion than the constitution. The constitution is determined by the dominant theme in terms of color, odor, sound, emotion, and purpose.

Three Treasures:
Protection, Enlightenment and Destiny

Frugality generates essence; compassion creates
vitality and mindfulness ... spirit.
The development of spirit requires refine-
ment guarding and penetration.
—Lao Zi

The three treasures model works for understanding wellness. Too often, Chinese medicine is conducted on a remedial basis, only correcting problems. It then is caught in the problem-reaction-solution bind. We must sometimes extricate ourselves from the mud of the complex sign-symptom matrix and attain a view, seeking that which is well.

The three treasures are *jing* (essence), *qi* (vitality), and *shen* (spirit). For the purposes of this book, I call them essence, vitality and spirit. In addition to wellness, they provide an excellent tool for exploring and treating constitution.

The vital life force flows through the channels protecting, transforming, holding, connecting and warming the body. Vitality commands blood via its movement through the vessels while holding bodily structures and consciousness upright. The mild warming nature of vitality catalyzes human interactions. In opposition to the stable holding function of vitality is its power to transform physiologically, personally, socially, and in terms of larger cosmological events.

Essence provides the foundation for both structure and function. This includes, but is not limited to the bones, central nervous system, and blood. They are all rooted within the kidneys. There are two types of essence: prenatal, which arrives with conception, and acquired, which is affected by lifestyle.

Conditions related to the prenatal essence tend to be present for as long as the patient can remember. The assessment rests within the strength of the bones and teeth or the strength and flexibility in the cartilage of the ears. The pulses of the left wrist are used to evaluate the prenatal essence while the right wrist is used to evaluate the status of the postnatal. Postnatal essence can be enhanced through lifestyle, herbs, and qi-gung. It primarily relates to good care of the body and the self.

The three treasures can be visualized through contemporary systems biology. The plant materials modulate the relationship between the central nervous system, endocrine system, and immune system in a form of psycho-neuro-immunology. The net result: plants affect how the individual responds to life and the decisions that are required. Thus, the movable karmas that are generated around decisions and actions begin to change.

Three classes of medicinals are defined in one of China's earliest herbals, the *Shen Nung Ben Cao*. Lowest grade agents are toxic. In the middle grade they have a direct action—opposing the psychological or physiological states. For example, if a person is in a fiery rage, use agents that purge fire such as Radix et Rhizoma Gentianae (*lóng dăn căo* 龙胆). The materials that alter karma are the superior class, and it is this arena where the materials that nourish the three treasures are located. They are often amphoteric, that is bi-directional, in their influence. This section provides tools for knowing which of the three treasures to emphasize when giving plant materials.

My favorite medicinal for the spirit is called reishi, or Ganoderma lucidum (*líng zhī* 灵芝). The character *líng* 灵 suggests that the people are seeking rain by the act of the shamans. It is the spiritual state of grace, whereby events fall right into place as one walks the path. Medicinals such as Astragalus membranaceus (*huáng qí* 黄芪)

in addition to other materials from the class of qi tonics in Chinese medicine. My favorite herb for essence—which has been with me since 1980—is Radix Polygoni multiflori (*hé shŏu wū* 何首乌).

Stories abound throughout the countryside of China and for millennia about *hé shŏu wū* 何首乌. They are similar and relate to the supplementation of essence. An ill, elderly, and alcoholic man stumbles in a drunken stupor. Discovering he can no longer stand due to the ravages of his disease, he finds his way to the ground for sleep. Upon awakening he discovers nearby, the *hé shŏu wū* plant and begins to eat its roots. Time passes, and he gradually regains his strength, is cured of alcoholism, finds meaningful work, becomes wealthy, gets married and has children. *Hé shŏu wū* supplements essence and blood, thereby providing a basis for self-esteem and essentially changing karma.

Embarking upon an exploration of herbal medicine, my world changed. I was living homeless, sometimes in a boarded area beside a house and sometimes in a van. It was an experiment about living on faith alone. This experiment, of course, was enhanced by the fact that there was no job or money. Yet grace came. Never was there a loss for food, study, resources, food, musical equipment, or as a musician, a place to practice. Just as these early stories of *hé shŏu wū*, which translates literally as Mr. He's black hair—I began eating the *hé shŏu wū*. That was 1980. I soon married, had children, went to school, and developed a career in Chinese medicine.

Assessment of the Three Treasures

The assessment of spirit is conducted by gazing at the eyes. Light refraction is assessed whether too dull or to bright, focused or unfocused. Neither should it be too intense.

Contemporary psychological theories of transference and counter-transference apply. Thus, we as practitioners note our own feelings and sensations, and to these we assign meaning. The developed practitioner's soma and psyche are fine-tuned instruments for understanding what takes place within the patient. These observations, however, must be verified through inquiry.

The assessment of vitality is by the flesh, and especially the cheeks and jaw line. Are the cheeks full or caved in? If the flesh is medium full, this is appropriate and the vitality is generally in good condition. Also, pay attention to the voice. Is it reasonably strong? Prognosis is improved when the cheeks are firm and full with reasonable amount of color while the voice of moderate strength.

Assess the essence by inspecting the integrity of the cartilage in the ears and by knocking upon bones. The ear cartilage should be firm and flexible. It is good if the ear lobe is long. One may inspect the teeth for the status of the bones. Tapping bone where available also assists the assessment of essence. The bones should be solid. It could be at the ankle, knee, wrist or elbow. Grasping the bone also tells the story of essence.

The three treasures can be evaluated using the pulses of the left wrist. The 1st (distal) position reveals spirit. The 2nd (middle) position is used to evaluate vitality. The 3rd (proximal) proximal position is used to evaluate essence and familial karmas.

There are general considerations for the evaluation of essence by pulse diagnosis. Root is imperative: if one feels pulse presence in the depth, there is root and therefore essence. If it gives way in the depth, there is a lack of essence for that organ. The pulse significating essence should therefore be felt in the depth and in the 3rd position. Essence may also be depleted if the whole left side is weak.

As for vitality—use force and amplitude of the pulse. The vitality may be weak if the pulse is deep, lacks force, or the whole right side is weak. It should be confirmed by a stellium of signs and symptoms that confirm depleted vitality such as a swollen tongue causing teeth marks or fatigue. Often symptoms are exacerbated with exertion when vitality is depleted.

When spirit is strong, the pulse is stable, yet responsive. When spirit is disturbed, the pulse may vibrate on the surface, it could change rate at rest, and it may be slippery in the left distal position, suggesting that phlegm "mists the mind." The dampness causes "brain fog." There are ways to discern the relations between the three treasures:

- If the spirit and essence are strong, with diminished vitality, it may be the result of lifestyle. Supplement the qi.
- When vitality and essence are strong, with diminished spirit, then consider spiritual problems or wrong actions weighing on the spirit. Supplement and clarify the spirit.
- If the spirit and vitality are strong, but the essence diminished, the problems this individual deals with are likely familial. With the spirit bright, but vitality and essence diminished, then the spirit is usurping the other treasures. It requires a change in action. This can be seen in someone like Jimi Hendrix who burned so brightly that the flame went out (Jarrett, 1999).

In addition to the evaluation of the three treasures, the organs that are involved in production of substances can be evaluated. The postnatal production of vitality and essence depends upon three physiological functions, acquisition of vitality from the air, food, and source root (lungs, digestion and endocrine function). This process generates blood, nutrient, and protective vitality. Consideration for production of vitality becomes important because it is one of the three treasures and combines with essence to provide a foundation for spirit. Further, the spirit is housed in the blood which is generated from the same process as vitality. Here we discuss tools for evaluating these substances and their production.

Evaluation of capacity for the upper, middle and lower to bring in air, food, and source vitality are critical to determine the etiology of deficiencies regarding the production of the three treasures. Simply compare the volume and force between the positions on the right wrist. The distal position relates to vitality acquired from the air. The middle position relates to vitality acquired from the food. The proximal position relates to the metabolic and essence vitality that contributes to the production of protective and nutrient vitality, vitality, and blood. The weakest position suggests the etiological culprit.

Daoist and alchemist Liu I Ming states, "The Sun, Moon, and stars are the three treasures of heaven, while essence, vitality, and spirit are the three treasures of humans. The Moon rules essence and *yin* fluids as a watery planet. The Sun rules vitality, particularly its *yang* fiery aspect. The stars rule the spirit as the consciousness of heaven" (Ming 1998)

Treasure	Cosmos	Depth	Weight	Dose	Plant Part	Position
Spirit	Stars	Superficial	Light	Small	Flowers, Laeaves	Distal
Vitality	Sun	Middle	Medium	Medium	Bark, Branches	Middle
Essence	Moon	Deep	Heavy	Large	Roots	Proximal

Table 2: Three Treasures, Pulse, Cosmology, and Herbs

Contemporary Notions of Self

Ideas about self are found scattered throughout the literature of early cultures. They are the roots of contemporary thought about self, ranging from atomistic, singular, and continuous views, to pluralized, multifaceted experiences self, of which the native only sees glimpses.

Integral theorist Allan Combs provides that, "We can think of the self as the subjective core of our conscious personality, the facet of ourselves most clearly identified with what we mean by 'I' or 'me'" (Combs 2002). He further suggests that, "We need to look more deeply into the self and realize that it is, in fact, more than our conscious sense of who we are… In other words, the self is a kind of self-organizing vortex at the center of the personality that sorts, organizes, and responds to the experiences the world brings us." From this vortex, self connects to others, mirroring back and forth, along the channels, pathways, or meridians, as described in Chinese medicine.

Postmodern social theorist Walter Truett Anderson describes the shifting landscape of identity as: *multiphrenia, proetean, de-centered or self-in-relation*. He uses the term *multiphrenia* to describe disparate voices of culture that define one's identity. It takes deep reflection to unbind one from these 'voices of the market place'. He uses the word *protean* to describe that self which changes to suit various circumstances. His notion of the *de-centered* being has no sense of self, but rather a flux constantly redefined and subject to change. Here, the subject does not speak language but rather is its creation. Having no enduring "I" we are what we are described to be. Through language and symbolic creations, we create each other and ourselves. Anderson's fourth term, *self-in-relation*, suggests that we live our lives, not as voices in the market place, nor as islands unto ourselves, but rather, we are in relation to people and cultural contexts. To rightly understand ourselves, we must understand our situation (Anderson 1997).

The experience of self, most often falters and balks, changing reality dependent upon context, when it does, the pulse changes. The nature of said pulse tells a secret about identity and identification within the moment.

Psychologist Carl Rogers creates a model that allows for an authentic sense of being (1961). This idealized notion of the singular self has generated a value of continuous and consistent expression of self across roles, responsibilities, and social contexts. The process of establishing social identity then becomes closely allied to the concept of the persona, which Goffman (1959) describes as "that part of the individual's performance, which regularly functions in a general and fixed fashion, to define the situation for those who observe the performance" (p. 22). The persona acts as the vehicle of standardization, allowing for others to understand the individual on the basis of projected character traits that have normative meanings. As a "collective representation," the persona establishes proper setting, appearance, and manner for the social role assumed by the actor, uniting interactive behavior with the personal front (p. 27). The actor, in order to present a compelling front, fills the duties of the social role and communicates the activities and characteristics of the role to other people in a consistent manner (Goffman 1959).

Rogers' concept of a "fully functioning organism" provides more depth than Goffman's view of the persona, where there is a direct knowledge of being, one that is free of, or at least able to minimize, the distortions of experience in awareness. Ideally, there is a full experience of all sensory and visceral reactions where the person accepts or learns to be the pattern—the underlying order—that exists in the ceaselessly changing flow of experience (Rogers 1961). Such authenticity creates fulfilling relationships.

Rogers claims in his book, *On Becoming a Person,* "Good communication, free communication, with or between people, is always therapeutic" (p. 330). If I can listen and understand concerns between one aspect of myself and another, I can use that information to reduce the distortions of meaning. This idea applies equally to conversations with others. If I can see an idea's personal meaning to another, if I can sense the emotional flavor that it has for that person, then potent forces of change may be released (p. 332).

The paradoxes between authentic and plural self begin to dissolve in what Jenny Wade calls "transcendent and unity stages of consciousness" (1996). Such a consistent state of being transcend the efforts toward an authentic and consistent positioning of the persona in arrayed social settings.

Yet, during neurotic moments, fragmented, anxious, disconnected parts of self arise and affect the experience. Mantras, prayer, ritual and breathing techniques help such conditions as do diet and herbs. There is a Daoist method of enhancing intrapersonal communications, called the smiling method, may be used to resolve this dilemma. The organs are asked to communicate with one another, smiling. Thus, from my heart, I smile at the liver, lungs, pancreas, and kidneys. From each of these organs, I smile at the others, listening to their voices. Thus, I find a harmonization of the patterns of self that emerge from the perspective of each of these organs. This "gestalt-like" communication poses new possibilities in the experience of self.

> "The self as understood by conventional knowledge exists and acts across time. If we analyze this understanding (which in itself "belongs" to the self), it appears that the self *establishes itself and the world that it knows* by moving off center, 'beyond' the point-instant of temporal knowledge. In one unified action, it *takes a position, posits a situation and imposes meaning.* The self finds itself in the world—its attention defines 'there' and 'then' and its vantage point locates 'here' and 'now'" (Tulku 1984, p. 147).

Wilhelm Reich was part of Sigmund Freud's inner circle in Vienna; however, the two parted ways as Reich began to develop his theories of social evolution. The split took place as radical sociologists influenced Reich, who considered the structure of society to mold the structure of the individual mind.

Reich considered mental illness to be much more prevalent than generally realized. Reich considered socio-political behaviors such as bigotry, prejudice, and fanaticism to be symptoms of a profoundly neurotic humanity. Reich labeled this illness of humanity as a major health problem and the *Emotional Plague of Mankind.* "This emotional plague accounts for war, crime, violence, rape, sadism, masochism, and almost everything that frightens about civilization" (Reich 1980b; Wilson 1987). Thus, individual conditions such as neuroses, psychoses, sociopathic behaviors, and their corresponding character armoring, rigid muscles and breathing correlate with the rigidity and armoring of society (1980a; 1980b).

Reich's bio-psycho-social views have influenced entire disciplines of body-mind centered therapies including Rolfing, and the Bioenergetics of Alexander Lowen (Lowen 1972; Painter 1987; Rolf 1989). The areas where Reich sees the *Emotional Plague of Mankind* arising are several: 1) mental conditions, including depression, anxiety, compulsion, phobia, perversion, and schizophrenia, 2) physical symptoms, such as asthma, cancer, ulcers, and sexual dysfunction, and 3) social problems, like war, violence, and crime. This emotional plague appears similar to the Chinese medical conception of qi stagnation, the mother of all disease.

Character armoring, rigidity, and blockage were seen by Reich to be the result of the past brutality of our species: not dissimilar to early Shang (ca. 1600 BC–ca. 1046 BC) and Zhou (ca. 1122 BC–ca. 256 BC) Dynasty conceptions of disease begat from the ancestors. There are no purely mental illnesses according to Reich.

METHODS OF TREATMENT

Pulse as a View into Soma and Psyche

*Objectivity is the delusion that observations
could be made without an observer.*
—Heinz von Foerster

Pulse diagnosis provides a view into the ways by which the person compensates for the events of life. As for constitution, the deep and proximal pulses both address as do the condition of the pulses on the left wrist. When the constitution is correctly identified and treated, many conditions and corresponding features of the pulse tend to self-correct.

The pulse is subjective and changeable, which is a good thing for our purposes. As a person recounts stories related to significant changes in their life, neurohumoral compounds in the blood are altered. The pulse changes in response, providing an exquisite tool for communication with deeper levels of the psyche. Essentially, the adaptive mechanisms are activated and one has a window into the ways in which an individual compensates during change and transformation.

The importance of recording the pulse while the patient discusses difficult life transitions should not be underestimated. Strategies developed from this knowledge address the underlying physiological response to change. The subjective knowledge arising under the fingers tell the story about the adaptations and compensations a person maintains as a response to the events of their life.

Trauma and the Eight Extraordinary Vessels

Infinity born to the wings of night, split by dawn
The weight of being crossed o'er the bone's wondering
—William Morris

The eight extraordinary vessels provide a scaffold for the treatment of trauma. They are the space that compensates for an extraordinary level of tragedy. As reservoirs, they speak directly to the profound resilience human beings express.

This chapter focuses upon birth trauma as an encapsulation of traumatic incidents that can take place through the course of life. Address of shock and trauma are necessary considerations in the complex diseases of humanity. Physical trauma affects the smooth flow of vitality and blood, with minor trauma affecting local flow and major trauma affecting the vitality and blood of the entire organism. Free flow reduction over time causes the heart to overwork and become taxed. This causes the local perfusion of nutrients and removal of waste materials to be affected, and that is the mere physical substrate, as below so above.

Wounds may recur during life transitions. Significant crises of life may loosen compensated states, thus bringing a person into contact with their core wounds and recurrent archetypal themes. These wounds are traumatic incidents around which the life narratives are built.

Trauma emerges recurrently as ecopsychosocial patterns over the course of life. Such conditions are well addressed through the tools of Chinese medicine. Acupuncture and herbal medicine alter the terrain in which these patterns have been bound in the individual throughout the musculoskeletal, endocrine, nervous, digestive, immune, and reproductive systems. Not limited to individual psyche, social surroundings of the individual include family, work and others in the environment also transform as the does the individual.

As children, adolescents, young adults and even as elderly, we make assumptions about reality. When accompanied by trauma, such impressions become mountains on the horizon of our lives. The stories we create at these times become the themes of our lives.

In early childhood, language develops in the context of magical thinking and imaginings that self is at the cause of events taking place. Thus, in response to criticism, the child builds language such as, "What is wrong with me?" During adolescence, this "self" languaging is built in the context of the teenager's social environment. Here the conversation becomes, "Why don't I fit in?" Finally, in young adulthood, the individual realizes that, "I'm on my own. It's up to me." The story at this stage relates to life purpose, mission, and livelihood. In the elder years, it may be, "what is my legacy?"

The problem with the assumptions made during these three stages is that—*we made them up*. Such creations disconnect us from the original self. This leads to the existential dilemma of depression, isolation, anxiety, and despair. These are problems that transform in the presence of another, whether that being is human or animal, plant, spirit—the solution is spiritual and conscious.

Birth Trauma

The pre and perinatal birth experience leaves imprints that are non-symbolic, nonverbal, non-logical, and imminently visceral. Few events overwhelm more than birth, leaving traces upon the individual, shaping and patterning the relationship between self and other, unconscious and conscious, personal and collective. This critical juncture of "pre and post heaven" forms a doorway through which myths and stories of our lives are made.

Gestational traumas are many and include: physical violence, sexual abuse, infections such as Fifth's disease, Streptococcus, HIV and AIDS, preeclampsia, toxemia, and recreational drugs such as alcohol, tobacco, and cocaine, malnutrition, psychosocial factors, antidepressant use during pregnancy, such as serotonin reuptake inhibitors (SSRIs), and pregnancy in older women.

As the birth takes place, further imprinting factors include: placenta previa, drugs, physical trauma including surgery, prematurity, Caesarian section, breech, cord around the neck, delayed birth, high forceps, and anesthesia. Similarly, events shortly after birth such as incubation, vaccination procedures, bright lights, and climate changes are all forms of trauma and shock that can affect in particular, the kidneys and heart from a Chinese medical point of view.

The complex emotional and biological events of birth become encapsulated, and may recur during significant transitions and transformations. These subsequent small deaths of change can bring about intense anxiety originating with survival threat and pain of birth. Aggression and rage seem to be a natural reaction to threat and prolonged frustration. This point of view links with Freud's understanding of depression as aggression turned against one's self.

A Brief History of Birth Trauma Concepts in the West

Otto Rank was the first to describe the effects of pre- and perinatal birth experiences upon the psychosocial states of the individual. He expanded upon Freud's statement, "All anxiety goes back originally to the anxiety at birth." Rank emphasized the birth experience as a determinant of mental life, its compulsions and its sicknesses. Rank was essentially the first to emphasize the importance of birth trauma on the development of the psyche and the corresponding life stories in his 1933 book, *The Trauma of Birth*. Ironically, Freud initially lauded Rank's work but changed his position due to the potential for Rank's theories to eclipse Freud's own Oedipal theory.

Rank's influence gained breadth, as his patient, Nandor Fodor, became a psychiatrist and focused on the formative experiences of birth, stating "In its shattering effect, birth can only be paralleled by death" (Fodor 1949). Francis Mott, a British patient of Fodor's, became a psychiatrist, writing on the mythological and dream content of prenatal life He was one of the first British psychiatrists to emphasize the effects of intrauterine life.

Frank Lake, Athanasios Kafkalides (1919–1989), and Stanislav Grof conducted research upon the enduring effects of gestational and perinatal experiences in adult life. Psychedelic psychotherapy, using LSD and other hallucinogenic drugs, provided the foundation for their work. Grof went on to formulate an extensive theoretical framework for the analysis of gestational and perinatal experiences, based on the four constructs he called Basic Perinatal Matrices.

Following the works of Wilhelm Reich (1897–1957), Lake and Grof each developed breathing techniques as an alternative to psychedelic drugs, which became subject to considerable legal difficulty since the 1960s. Similarly, Leonard Orr (born 1937) spawned a popular movement amongst the laity called Rebirthing Breathwork.

Birth Trauma Intensity

In his theory of regressive therapy, Frank Lake organizes thought about birth trauma into four categories of intensity. First, there is an ideal state, relatively pain-free, involving no significant trauma, where forward movement takes place relatively unimpeded. This "good" birth results in an optimistic life where challenges are overcome.

The second level of birth trauma intensity relates to difficult dilation. The pelvis, too narrow for the head to pass through, often reshapes the cranium. Suffering takes place over a longer period of time than in level one. As a result of this manageable stress, the birthed infant desires a return to the comfortable womb. The events are bearable and strengthen the person as it evokes effective and non-neurotic defenses.

The third stage involves resistance to pain so intense that coping mechanisms begin to falter and repression takes place. In the third stage, "the head is jammed in the pelvis and can move neither forwards nor backwards. The will to return to the womb is as useless as the will to move forward. Only one struggle is possible, the struggle to live in spite of growing distress, crushing of the head, and lack of oxygen. The identity if someone suffering from an anxiety state not uncommonly has this biological emergency as its primary determinant" (1978a).

Lake calls the fourth category "transmarginal stress," where the pain is so powerful that the person cuts off completely from the real self and may even turn against it, seeking death. "The loathing of the pain of being born may be so great that the wish to die almost entirely replaces the former longing to live. In fact, the intensity of the earlier longing is transformed, mechanically and without any act of the will to the latter, at the point where sheer intolerance of pain takes over" (1978a).

Arthur Janov, the originator of primal therapy, suggests hope in that those who relive the perinatal death experience seem to resolve fixations on death and suicide. In this thinking, the moments surrounding birth determine whether or not one will consider suicide as a serious alternative at a later age. In his theory, suicidal acts are an attempt to return to the death feeling, a way of recovering the original physiological experience where the baby came close to death in order to live (Janov 1970).

Perinatal Matrices of Stanislov Grof

Psychiatrist Stanislov Grof investigated birth trauma and developed a scaffold upon which to hang knowledge about the birth process. Parsing the birth experience into four stages, he called it the "perinatal birth matrix" (Grof 1975). The research was originally performed prescribing LSD. Grof now uses breathing techniques to elicit the birth experience.

The birth matrix may be applied to circumstances beyond the individual, including social, biological, and cosmological systems. The gestational phase connects with a stable Garden of Eden stage, where "normalization" takes place in the form of a plateau. As the "natural flow of events" progress, stagnant weather fronts emerge, tectonic plates get stuck, and crowds become frustrated. The contraction phase happens. During the thrusting phase, there can be volcanic activities, violent demonstrations, and supernovae. Lastly, there is the exit phase, where new freedoms are found, including the acceptance of disappointment as a Promethean bind forms the new cycle.

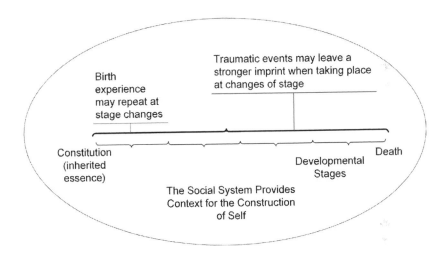

Figure 1: Chronology of Life Stages and Imprints

This map of "Self" presents the stages and imprints. Psychological Dynamics in the Transformation of the Individual—Time as Stages and or Phases in Life.

Birth matrices are general experiential patterns correlated to the stages of birth and, according to Grof, do not imply a causal nexus. The gestational stage correlates with the peaceful and harmonious ecstasy of the oceanic type, a spiritual type of ecstasy, tension-free egoless identification with the Universe and God, with essential qualities of love, light, and security. This matrix relates to the original condition of the intrauterine existence during which the child and his mother form a symbiotic unity. Unless some noxious stimuli interfere, the conditions for the child are optimal, involving security, protection appropriate milieu, and satisfaction of all needs. This symbiotic unity can have both a disturbed and an undisturbed nature (1985).

During the contractions, feelings of antagonism with mother occur during the first clinical stage of delivery. The fetus, mechanically and chemically alienated from the mother, has no possibility of immediate escape, which may later manifest as feelings of being trapped, of being hopelessly caught and overwhelmed. This episode belongs, perhaps, to the worst experiences a human being can have. Clinical symptoms correlated with this stage during psychotherapeutic sessions with entheogenic substances, include general motor inhibition, agonizing mental pain and suffering, anxiety, overwhelming feelings of guilt and inadequacy, absolute lack of zest, selectively negative perception of the world and one's own life, black-and-white perception of the world without colors, and feelings of an unbearable and inescapable life situation with no hope of any solution. Also, the physical manifestations of depression are in agreement with this concept: feelings of oppression and constriction, loss of appetite and rejection of food, retention of urine and feces, inhibition of libido, headaches, cardiac distress, subjective breathing difficulties and various physical complaints interpreted occasionally in a hypochondriacal way. The suicidal ideation of this condition has typically the form of a wish not to exist, to fall into a deep sleep, forget everything, and not to awake the next day. It would connect with the Freudian model as episodes of early oral frustration in infancy, emotional deprivation in infancy and childhood, and various traumatic events in which the subject played the role of passive victim (Grof 1975).

As the infant is thrust through the birth canal, synergism with the mother occurs during the second clinical stage of delivery. The uterine contractions continue, but the cervix stands wide open, and the gradual and difficult propulsion through the birth canal begins—an enormous struggle for survival, mechanical crushing pressures, and high degree of suffocation. The system, then no longer closed, presents the possibility: termination of the unbearable appears. The third stage of "Death-Rebirth Struggle" takes place when tremendous force on the fetus expels it from the womb. The mother's womb, which for many months was experienced as a loving, benign, and heavenly environment, has turned into an atmosphere of titanic force where the young fetus negotiates life and death. The experiences of the third matrix are intensely dramatic, ominous, heavy, and place one's self (or the collective) in immense struggles usually involving the status quo versus chaos and destruction. These can often be intensely violent times, or they can illuminate a tremendous struggle without any sense of resolution. Grof describes the third perinatal stage: "Perhaps the most striking aspect of this matrix is the atmosphere of titanic struggle, frequently of catastrophic proportions ... The experiences can reach a painful intensity that exceeds by far what it seems any human could possibly bear" (Grof 1993).

When separation from the mother occurs, the symbiotic union ends, and a new relationship with the mother must occur during the third clinical stage of delivery. In this matrix, the agonizing experiences of several hours culminates, the movement through the birth canal is completed, and a sudden relief and relaxation follow the maximum intensification of tension and suffering. The fourth birth stage experience, as described by Grof, illustrates the resolution to the titanic conflict that the fetus has undergone. The fetus, released from the tremendously potent contractive forces of the womb, births into a new universe, a new existential situation. The newborn child is liberated from the contractive pulsations of the womb that seemed like an onslaught of monstrously destructive energy. Here, the child experiences a sense of liberation and relief. As Grof describes, "This new situation is a significant improvement over the previous two stages ... A person who has overcome the enormous trials of the second and third matrices and is enjoying the experience of rebirth associated with the fourth matrix usually has triumphant feelings" (Grof 1993).

I have explored the application of Grof's theory in the clinic and classroom since listening to him in 1995. It was not until I entered a program in transformative studies at California Institute of Integral Studies in 2007 that I realized this four-stage process, described as a perinatal birth matrix, tends to recur during the rebirths that take place during developmental stage transitions and significant life changes.

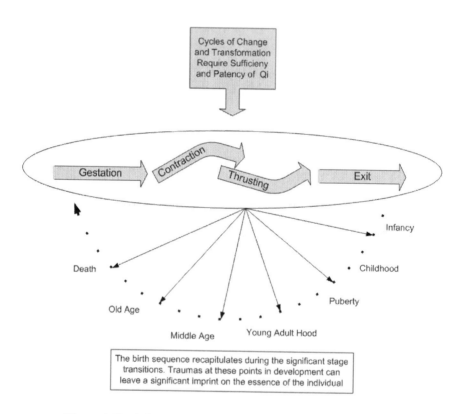

Figure 2: Birth Stages as Recurrent Themes in Life Transitions

Grof's theory of the perinatal birth matrix fits in the moment between stages of development, as discussed by theorists Piaget

(1960), Gillian (1993) and Kohlberg (1981). It would appear that Grof's perinatal birth matrix can be applied to transitional moment and transformational phenomena, rather than the stages where "plateaus" occur. Consider one's job, where, after initial entry, it can be associated with the gestational phase, relatively peaceful and productive. As dissatisfaction emerges, one creates stories that support the irritations and stagnations. Depression and irritability can ensue. Then one begins to push in order to create an environment for change. Reasons for leaving are created and eventually separation can be accomplished.

Perinatal Set		Postnatal Set	
Du	SI3	Yang qiao	UB62
Ren	Lu7	Yin qiao	K6
Dai	Gb41	Yang wei	SJ5
Chong	Sp4	Yin wei	P6

Table 3: Correlations with Grof's Perinatal Birth Matrix

Pulse and Birth Trauma

The events of birth leave imprints upon the neurovascular and other parts of the circulatory system. In as much as the upper regions of the head, neck, extremities and pulmonary system are affected, the signs of trauma can be palpated in distal pulse positions. Hammer describes the distal position pulses as inflated, flat, or bird pecking. There may also be arrhythmias. Breach birth can cause the pulse to be inflated (tense and full quality). When the cord is wrapped around the neck, the pulse can be flat (2001). Under these conditions, a rough pulse is another possibility.

The impact of birth trauma is a physiological as well as a psychological event that leaves traces upon the pulse. When a condition begins during parturition or at birth, the proximal positions tend to be deep or weak, suggesting kidney *yang* essence depletion. A detailed history should be taken so as to rule out postnatal events as the cause for any of the signs or symptoms. A bluish-green tinge around the mouth suggests that the circulatory function was affected during the birthing process, as can a retreated, misanthropic timber (Hammer 2001). As a prelude to the next section, gestational trauma may lead to a level pulse at the middle depth. Trauma during the contraction phase may lead to a pulse that is full in the middle positions compared to the distal and proximal. During the thrusting phase, trauma may lead to a deep pulse. Trauma postpartum may lead to a pulse that is level and superficial (Morris, 2002).

All traumatic events affect both heart and circulation. If appropriate, employ treatment strategies such as open orifices, move blood, and vitality in order to resolve old traumatic events. The combination of aromatic open orifice agents and blood stasis dispelling agents can have a profound spiritual impact and resolve deep-seated trauma of the past.

I learned to use *Yu Nan Bai Yao* from Leon Hammer and John H.F. Shen. They used it as an herbal protocol. I have used it one to two hours prior to stimulating the appropriate points in order to enhance the efficacy of treatment. This formula used to be secret, posing ethical problems in the west for prescription. The ingredients are now published, making this a reasonable option for the qualified herbalist.

Perinatal Trauma and the Eight Extraordinary Vessels

As an expression of the number 8, infinity of possibilities may be treated through these extraordinary vessels. The *Nan jing* states in Difficulty 27, "the eight extra vessels are used to prevent flooding during storms." Such a flood relates to neurohumoral chemicals that overwhelm the individual during traumatic events leaving an imprint that can be triggered by various sensory input such as odors, sounds, images, and sensations. These triggers can be called n-grams by Scientologists or samskaras in the Hindu traditions. Materially, these are neural pathways that have created patterns or grooves in the structure and physiology of the brain in such a way that they are habituated and easily triggered. These are the materials of posttraumatic stress syndrome. The acupuncture vessels of the *du*, *yang wei*, and *yang qiao* all have pathways around and through the brain. The nuclear vessels all have a root within the life gate and the kidneys, thus they have a relationship to the brain in terms of the marrow relationship of the kidneys.

The eight extraordinary vessels are often used as a direct means of modulating the neurohumoral and endocrinological responses to stressful events. The *yin qiao* can be used to treat habituated neurohumoral responses to stress. Often called a "trauma treatment," any of the extraordinary vessels may be used based upon the presenting signs and symptoms. Rote use of a single channel or point for a specific condition without a systemic view that takes into account the whole picture will not be as effective. Pulse diagnosis provides a reliable indicator of an active and compensating extraordinary vessel.

I relate the four primal vessels to the four phases of perinatal experience. These connections are the *ren* with the oceanic womb state, the *dai* with the contraction phase, the *chong* with thrusting phase, and the *du* with the exit phase. The coupled vessels of the *yin* & *yang qiao*, *yin* & *yang wei* are related to postnatal traumatic events that push one to the edge of existence. The eight extras relate to deeper reservoirs that the twelve main channels rely upon to prevent physiological and psychological flooding when the storms of life become too intense. There are few events in life more overwhelming than birth and death. The infant's descent through the birth canal follows the pathway of the Eight Extraordinary vessels as they emerge from within the life-gate toward the perineum in order, *ren-dai-chong-du*.

The oceanic experience of the womb connects deeply with the *ren mai*. The contracting phase fits perfectly with the function of the *dai mai* during labor. Traumatic events occurring at the *dai mai* (contraction) stage can cause the individual to feel blocked and obstructed in life, according to Grof's theorem. The *dai mai* can be used to effectively suppress unwanted feelings. The thrusting stage shares the same name of the *chong*. Pelvic thrusts can bring on volcanic, eruptive pushing in order for the child to exit the birth canal. There may be meconium and blood as intensity peaks. The *chong mai* shares the blood component in that it can be considered to be the abdominal aorta. The *du* channel runs right up the spine, and the child exiting the birth canal has autonomy consistent with sea of *yang*, the *du* vessel.

The Four Birth Stages and Nuclear Vessels

1. The oceanic womb state relates to the *ren mai*.
2. The contractions begin under the influence of the *dai mai*.
3. The baby drops into birth canal under the influence of the *chong mai*.
4. The baby comes out relying on itself under the influence of the *du mai*.

Life changes can recapitulate the birth process. Take for examples, the teenager preparing to leave home. Prepuberty provides for a mild and relatively content state of affairs consistent with the gestational stage. As the hormonal changes begin to take place with puberty, there can be frustration, depression, feelings of entrapment, and an essential blocking of the will. At some point, this erupts into the 3rd matrix at the thrusting stage when the emotions become more cataclysmic and the energy increases so separation from the parents can be realized. Upon leaving home, the youngster often feels the same levels of freedom and birth that correlate with stage four, the exit phase of Grof's perinatal birth matrix.

Pulse Assessment of the Eight Extraordinary Vessels

The following pulse images do not necessarily indicate vessel pathology; they indicate activity. The body compensates and adapts using the eight extra vessels. Given an appropriate confirmation, the presence of these pulses signal useful interventions. The four nuclear vessels of the *du, dai, ren,* and *chong* are the primary correlations for analysis of the imprint left by the perinatal experience. Hold the patient's pulse while they discuss their birth experience, either what they can recall or what they have heard from their mother or other persons present at the birth.

The master couple extensions of the *yin & yang wei, yin & yang qiao* are more suggestive of postnatal adaptations to events. The *yin & yang qiao* tend to be activated in response to musculoskeletal and physical trauma. The *yin* and *yang wei* tend to be activated in response to psychosocial traumatic incidents.

Place the fingers on either the left or right wrist (take care that the fingers are even with even pressure). Press until the first impulse hits the fingers. If all fingers touch the vessel simultaneously and superficially hit at once at the qi depth, consider it a *du mai* pulse. A *ren* pulse is level in the middle depth. If the pulse is deep, it suggests a *chong mai* pulse. The *chong* pulse may not be level. The *chong mai* can be forceful, changing force, or uneven between the positions.

During initial pressing stage, if the index finger touches the pulse first, consider a *yang qiao* pulse. If the middle finger touches first, a *dai* pulse. If the third finger hits first, a *yin qiao* pulse.

To locate a *yang wei* pulse, one must roll the index finger toward the radius. If the pulse extends such that as one rolls the finger over the radius and the pulse can still be felt, this suggests a *yang wei* pulse. It must be confirmed by rolling toward the ulna in the 3rd position. This is the most reliable method for discerning the transverse placement of the *yang wei* pulse. The reverse is true for the *yin wei* pulse. The first sign to look for: an ulnar displacement of the radial artery in the 1st position. Achieve confirmation by a radial distortion of the proximal or 3rd position. The *yin & yang wei* vessels tend to be related to postnatal events of the psychosocial persuasion. For exploring birth trauma, we are primarily interested in those vessels that relate to perinatal experience, the core nuclear vessels.

Group 1: is long and level across the distal, middle, and proximal positions. The *du* pulse is superficial, long, and level. The *ren* pulse is at a middle depth, long, and level. The *chong* pulse is deep throughout, yet often uneven.

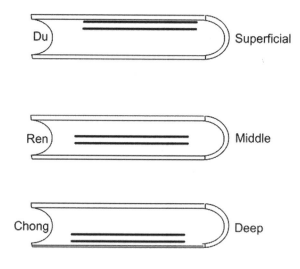

Figure 3: Ren, Du, and Dai Pulses

Group Two: The *yin qiao* is larger in the *yin* position (proximal—*chǐ*). The *yang qiao* is larger in the *yang* position (distal—*cùn*). The *dai* is larger in the middle (*guān*) suggesting accumulation in the *dai* or belt channel. When pressing, the first position to arrive under the fingers defines the image.

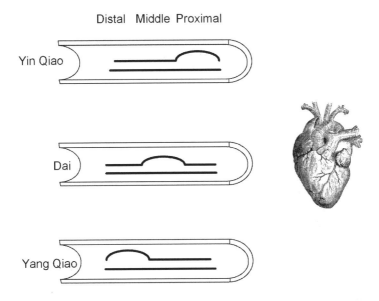

Figure 4: Yin Qiao, Yang Qiao, and Dai Pulses

Group Three: In the distal position, the *yang wei* vessel is displaced toward the *yang* (thumb—radial) and the *yin wei* is displaced toward the *yin* (little finger—ulnar). This must be confirmed in the proximal position by opposite displacement so that a true diagonal line is present. The *yin wei* and *yang wei* pulse descriptions are the only discussion of vessel displacement in current English translations of classical and neoclassical literature.

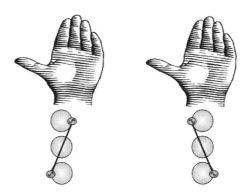

Figure 5: Yin Wei and Yang Wei Pulses

When a case begins to present life patterns and symptoms that correlate with one of the perinatal birth matrices, a single vessel usually dominates the picture. The master point for the vessel can be used along with tender points along the trajectory of the extraordinary vessel. Having the patient breathe with the diaphragm in a full abdominal breathing method improves outcomes.

Matrix	I	II	III	IV
Humor	Phlegmatic	Melancholic	Sanguine	Choleric
8 Extra Nuclear Channels	Ren	Dai	Chong	Du
Herbal categories	Nourish yin	Boost vitality	Nourish blood	Boost yang
Points	Lung 7	GB 41	Spleen 4	SI 3
Shen's Systems	Organ	Digestive	Circulatory	Nervous
Pulse	Level at Blood depth	Excess Middle Burner	Organ depth	Floating Level
Kingdom	Mineral	Plant	Animal	Human
Hindi	Hiranyagarba	Brahma	Shiva-Kali	Vishnu
Christianity	Teachings Garden of Eden	Desert, expulsion from the Garden	Crucifixion	Rebirth
Culture	Pygmies (paradise)	Totalitarianism Concentration Camps	Revolution Overthrow	End of war celebration parades
Miasm	Petroleum	Syphilitic	Sycotic	Psoric

Table 4: Master Points and Prenatal—Postnatal Vessel Groupings

Along with the use of an extraordinary vessel, the periumbilical points of tenderness and stagnation can be used to reinforce the connection with the bi will rth process as it relates to the severance of the umbilical cord, thus creating the first scar. The point of final severance takes place at the umbilicus. From the prenatal state, it links directly to the *du*, the *ren*, and the *chong*. Palpate for stagnations here to address perinatal trauma along with the appropriate nuclear vessel.

Spirit, Consciousness, and Pulse Diagnostic Methods

The world must move my heart but to the heart's discovery of its self.
—W.B. Yeats

A Method for Assessing the Spirit

There is a tendency in human interactions to assign meaning based upon assumptions rather than describe events. Such a condition poses distinct problems throughout life in general and the clinic in particular. Stress and anxiety are words that highlight this problem. In order to generate clarity, rather than compounding my assumptions upon those the patient makes when a patient reports anxiety, I ask where they feel their concern bodily. I ask what the word anxiety means to them since the meanings are so diffuse in popular use, so much so as to become useless in the clinical context. We must discover that which is closer to the real.

Behaviorist B.F. Skinner and psychiatrist Milton Erickson know that when they ask people what they perceive, they are more likely to get assumptions and interpretations rather than a sensory report of experience (Keeney 2011). A pathway to such knowledge emerges when I inquire as to what is actually being experienced in the body. This will lead to a more connected treatment. Similarly, when observing the pulse, we are involved with abstractions; that is, we must take the sensations and convert them into descriptive language. This language should first be descriptive of the sensations, rather than interpretive, in order to maintain a cognitive process, which is closer to the real.

Here we controvert the assumption of describing events materially and then assigning meaning. Rather, in this method, we take the meanings assigned by the directions and apply them to the pulse, such that when it conforms, it can be used to direct action.

Pulse diagnosis of the spirit takes place in the distal left position, which correlates with the heart, the "house of spirit." For these reasons, this location is where we begin the initial inquiry into the nature of spirit disturbance. I use what I call the "compass method" for this purpose.

The "compass method" has roots in the chapter from *The Yellow Emperor's Classic* titled "Internal Medicine Classic of Collected Truths," where physician Qi Bo states: Within the *cùn* [right distal] position, there is the division of superficial and deep levels, the proximal and distal positions and the left and right sides. The essential (of determining) vacuity or repletion, life or death all lie within the *cùn* opening (Wang 1997, p. 23). Ming Dynasty (1368–1644 C.E.). Physician Li Zhi Zhen also addressed the four directions in both diagnostics and therapy, "… in the radial pulses, *yin* and *yang* communicate and meet, for within there are five divisions, front, back, left and right, which each govern their correspondences" (Li 2006, Chapter 17, Line 1).

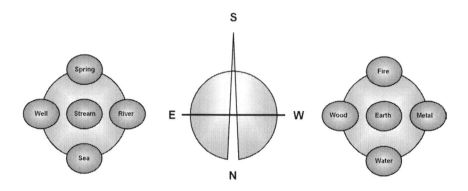

Figure 6: Directional Positions, Transformations, and Spirits

Now that we have classical authority for the technique, let us explore a creative application to contemporary practice. We apply the method to the left distal position as a tool for assessing the condition of spirit with respect to the transformations and the directions. Use the compass method in the left distal position and roll the finger into each of the directions. The fullest direction indicates the active aspect of the *shén* 神. The patient's left indicates *hún* 魂, distal—*shén* 神, right—*pò* 魄, center—*yì* 意 and proximal—*zhì* 志. Each of these spirits lives in its respective organ:

- The spirit which resides in the liver, the hún 魂, belongs to the East. It is located in the left or radial aspect of the heart position (left distal). The hún aspect of self has transcendental, dream time features.

- The spirit which resides in the lungs, the pò 魄, belongs to the West. It is located in the right or ulnar aspect of the heart position (left distal). The pò aspect of self is incarnating and presencing, it seeks to experience the world through the senses and the 7 orifices.

- The yì 意 thinks. It creates possibilities and can worry. It is the spirit, which resides in the spleen/pancreas and is located in the center of the pulse, located in the left or radial aspect of the heart position (left distal)

- The zhì 志 intends. Arriving in the north, this aspect of will is evaluated in the proximal aspect of the pulse, located in the left or radial aspect of the heart position (left distal).

- We have discussed shén 神 extensively. As a singular expression, it reflects pure conscious being as a unity field. In this context, it belongs to the south and the heart.

Rolling the index finger in each direction permits discovery of the dominant sensation. Place the index finger in the superficial component of the waveform in the left distal position (*cùn* or 1st position). Follow the surface, maintaining contact—this is the path of the pulse. After rolling in each direction, I find the fullest sector; it indicates a possible involvement of that spirit.

If the dominant sensation is in the radial aspect of the left distal position (left part of the heart position), then go to the position for the liver: the left middle position. The compass is then performed there in order to understand which transformation is out of balance within the liver and which is causing the *hún* to be disturbed. If the liver position (left middle) is most full distally, this correlates with fire. Thus, there is a fire disturbance in the house of the *hún*. We, therefore, treat the fire point on the liver channel, Liver 2 (*xíng jiān* 行间).

As another example, if the left distal position extends or presents fullness to the patient's right, explore the lungs in the right distal position. Accomplish this by performing the compass method in the right distal position. This will result in a single point that adjusts the lungs as a house of the *pò*, the incarnating aspect of spirit.

If the left distal position extends distally, consider it to be fire and your assessment is complete. You will perform treatment upon the fire point on the heart or pericardium channels, Heart 8 (*shào fǔ* 少府) or Pericardium 8 (*láo gong* 劳宫).

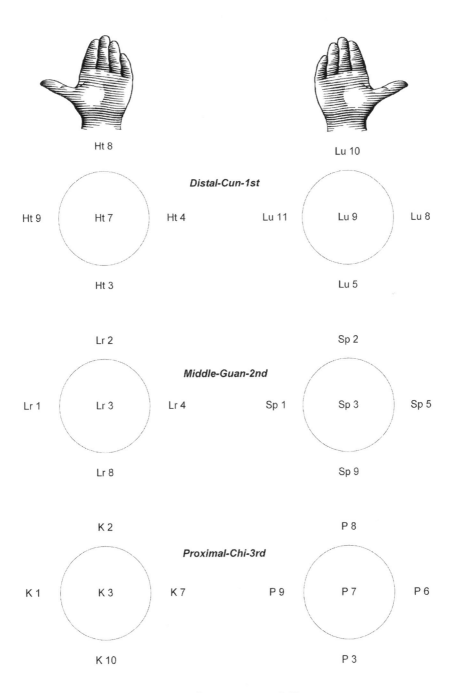

Figure 7: Point Associations with Directions

Case Vignette One

Mary entered our clinic clearly able to function in life. Her clothes were need, she was able to communicate with the front desk people effectively, and her interactions with the interns were socially appropriate. She described having fallen and hurt her arm. The cause of which, however, was being "struck by ghosts". Ghostly disturbances, may be considered a problem of spirit. And in many cultures are considered to be a part of life. Given her capacity for normal social interaction, we did make a referral to a mental health professional for the problem. Rather, we considered her condition to be squarely at the center of certain premodern Chinese thought. Since the heart is the house or throne of spirit, we palpate it for heart position in the four directions as well as the center. The pulse was distorted in the direction of metal, that is, to her right. This suggests a disturbance of the pò 魄. We therefore direct our attention towards the house of the pò, the lungs. Placing only the index finger upon the right distal position we palpate in all four directions and the center. The pulse is more full in the proximal direction. This suggests an imbalance of water within the lungs and the element of metal. The technique is one of correspondences. We therefore treat the water point on the lung channel. As we do so, the distracted and anxious look in her eyes darting around hypervigilant checking each person out of the room homes down to a steady presence in herself. The anxiety about the ghost that attacked her and cause the fall sides are concerns are alleviated and her spirit becomes stabilized. This is reaffirmed in the following visit where she exudes gratefulness for having cleared the problem as she perceived it.

My students and I have been using this method for treating patients with borderline personality disorders, bipolar disorders, depression, anxiety, and suicidal ideations. Some of these patients report experiences with ghosts. Such conditions should be referred to the appropriate professional. Chinese medicine provides a useful tool in the care of such conditions. All of these patients demonstrate *shen* disturbance. These patients may have an unstable gaze and affected speech, where ideas are unclearly communicated and hurried or slurred. After treatment with this method, the patient feels connected, heard, and that their problem has been addressed. The gaze gains some luminosity, stability, and presence, and they have a smile.

The plural and unified self are visibly apparent in the luminous glow of the eyes. The integrated self has a clear and singular refraction, clear and stable. The points that relate to the organs where the spirits reside can be mapped in a way that organizes and harmonizes the various forms of self. The *shen* pulse method provides a way of weaving the spirit together in harmony.

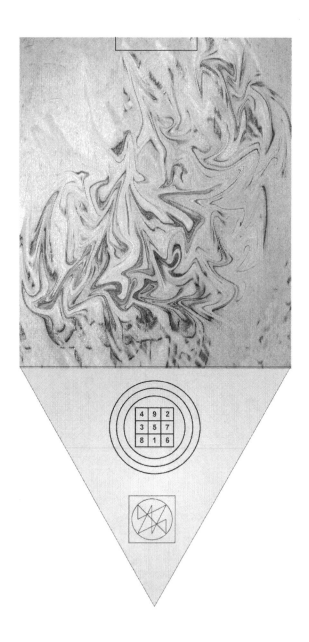

PROFECTION METHODS

Profection: Time and Space Intersections

Early cultures divide circles—representing the whole—by various numbers. The number five is commonly used to describe repentance, transformation, and types of people. Along with the primary channels of acupuncture, the twelve-fold division of the circle is also used to describe the day, year, and developmental stages in an individual's life, from childhood to teen years to young adulthood, midlife, and career culmination.

Profection is a Greek term for the practice of locating a moment in time and assigning meaning to it. Here, we use it to locate a moment in the past according to the channel that was active at that point in time (Valens 2004). Thus, the *profection* in this practice can be characterized as a *chronotope*, which is the intersection between space and time.

A *chronotope* describes a spatial-temporal matrix governing the base condition of personal and collective narratives. This can also include the intersection of process and form as an imprint upon the physical structures, such as the face or any body segment, as a sign of historical events.

The *chronos*, or a moment in time, is located upon the *topos* a location in space. This can be a circular form such as the umbilicus or the eye. It can also be employed over any long bone such as the femur, radius, or fibula. In this instance, the narrative includes the description of acupuncture points as representative of the intersection of time and space. We find it in the correlations between the seasons, times of day, and the five transformations. Therefore, the wood points and channels are active in spring, and fire points and channels are active in summer.

The experience of time can be conceived as a connected set of experiences (Bergson 1960). Since the clock has a circular format, it correlates with the sun moving along the plane of the ecliptic. The ecliptic is the band of stars that are eclipsed as the sun passes between where we stand and the ability to visualize the stars that are beyond the sun. The circle symbolizes boundary and enclosure, completion, and returning cycles (Fraser 1986). A whole segment of time or space can be divided into twelve. In this instance, we use the correlation with the twelve channels.

The umbilicus forms the center. It sits at the core of the human experience and extends to the environs wherein they operate. This first scar becomes a poignant circle wherein one may access the whole of life experience in the context of both space and time.

In terms of systemic physiology, significant events leave a lasting impression upon the neurotransmitter pathways and consequently, the central nervous system stores them as memories. The patterns recur throughout physiological systems shaping the homeodynamics locally and systemically. The local impact takes place in terms of the limbic, endocrine, neurovascular, and other functional components related to the autonomic nervous system. We know that lifestyle can imprint upon the genomics of an individual as we now know that epigenetic phenomena can now imprint upon the RNA-DNA code. The profection provides a tool for connecting to and transforming these phenomena by connecting to the location in time of a particular event in the past. Thus, the impact of trauma is manifold—from the center and throughout the complexity of physiological systems.

Profection Method

This method treats people who suffer from an event with a specific year of onset, be it spiritual, emotional, social, mental, or physical.

The profection may be used to target the current year or to access a year in the life when a certain event occurred. This could be the onset of disease or a major event that affected decisions that an individual makes about their life.

The practice involves factoring out twelve in order to identify the active channel at the time of a trauma. To do this, divide the age by twelve, take the remainder, and count forward from the lung channel along the organ clock, assigning a year per channel. Each cycle begins with the lung channel and moves through the sequences. If it is before age one, then the liver channel is considered.

The organ clock is set over the umbilicus from the patient's perspective. Thus, the Large Intestine channel is at the patient's left at nine o'clock. The pericardium is at the patient's right in the three o'clock position. Directly superior to the umbilicus is the Heart channel. Directly inferior to the umbilicus is the Gallbladder Channel. Again, counting from the lung the location upon the umbilicus is identified for a significant life-changing trauma.

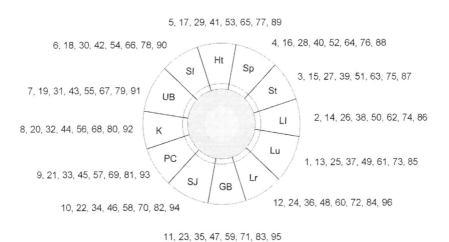

Figure 8: Organ Clock with Corresponding Ages

At approximately ½ *cùn* away from the umbilicus, the needle is inserted at a 45-degree angle toward the root. The tip of the needle just touches the scar tissue. This is the appropriate depth. There is no need to penetrate into the scar tissue, bringing about further trauma.

Caution is in order and cannot be overemphasized. This procedure requires informed consent. Connecting to a traumatic moment in the past can be very difficult. I have seen patients exhibit various forms of catharsis from catatonia to shaking vibratory states.

It is important, therefore, to activate the adaptive capacity of the eight extraordinary vessels (8EV). The pulses of these eight extraordinary vessels should be evaluated after placing the profected point. The 8EV image that arises upon needling the umbilical area that relates to the channel of the profected year and directs to the vessel that can be treated. It is important that the extraordinary vessels are employed in conjunction with the profection in order to assist resolving the materials that arise during and after the profection treatment. More importantly: gently seek permission and proceed only when safe!

Take the age of your patient at a peak moment. It can be traumatic or enlightening. Factor out 12, subtract 12 over and over until there is a remainder. Then, count channels beginning with the lung. Use Table 5 for convenience:

By Circuit		Organ Clock in Sequence of Channels		
1st Circuit	1. Lu	2. LI	3. St	4. Sp
2nd Circuit	5. Ht	6. SI	7. UB	8. K
3rd Circuit	9. Pc	10. SJ	11. GB	12. Lr

Table 5: Organ Clock and Circuit Relationships of the Channels

After factoring out 12 from the age of an incident, count from the lung channel to the channel of the profection. Place the image of an organ clock over the umbilicus (please see Figure 8). The image is adjusted for the right directions. Under the segment that corresponds with a year of trauma, there should be some palpable stagnation.

Case Vignette One

This case is an example of using the profection for the current year. A 27-year-old woman named Scotty had a crisis of life purpose. Common themes at this stage of life involve decisions about what one will and will not choose to do as a mission. Thus, the stage relates strongly to maturation. She also reported a high degree of emotional lability.

Since the stage development-related emotional distress was happening at the moment, I profected her age to 27. Dividing 28 by 12, leaves 4. Counting from the lung channel as 0, and around the organ clock, Lu-LI-St-Sp ... leads to the spleen as the 4th channel for the profection of her 27th year. I placed the organ clock over her naval and pressed toward the root of the umbilicus where a lumpy stagnation was palpated and presented with tenderness.

I decided to focus on earth and, since it was a developmental stage concern, to use the eight extraordinary vessels. For earth, this would be the *chong*, which has Sp4 (*gōng sūn* 公孙) as the master point and other points, such as St30 (*qì chōng* 气冲) and lower abdominal kidney points. The emotional state involved "crying at the drop of a hat." As a result, I decided to employ a divergent channel treatment. Because the theme was earth, I selected the stomach channel divergent, using the *he*-sea point St36 (*zú sān lǐ* 足三里, the window of the sky point St9 (*rén yíng* 人迎), and Du 20 (*bǎi huì* 百会).

The patient practices acupuncture and has extensive experience receiving acupuncture treatments. She reported an extraordinary experience compared to her other treatments. She said that she could feel the vitality oscillating laterally and then vertically. She also reported becoming emotionally stable and centered after the treatment.

Profection treatments can be repeated; the benefits, however, have limits and can only be repeated so much in a given time frame. Treatment with acupuncture ideally takes the weather, stage of life, season, time of day, constitution, and variables of the history and physical into consideration for the construction of the treatment. An effective treatment can be repeated, but sensitivity to the changes in these variables should also be employed.

The profection happens in the context of all other models of care, and in the moment, and over time, but when etiology connects to current events, the profection can be especially useful.

Case Vignette Two

Mary had Parkinson's, a degenerative disease of the nervous system thought to have no cure. She believed the Parkinson's disease was triggered by a brown recluse spider bite years ago that had then progressed to kidney failure for which she had to go on short-term dialysis. Whether the spider bite contributed to the development of Parkinson's or not, we used that date for a profection. This led to improvement, and her speech was more articulate and her gate improved.

The students had begun needling the scar from the spider bite, which I had encouraged. It occurred to me three weeks ago, as I walked into the room and the interns stood around in their white coats, trying to figure out what to do next, that we could use the organ clock and use the profection method to connect to the year of the spider bite. I divided by twelve with four remaining. I then counted from the lung to the large intestine to the stomach to the spleen. Sure enough, there was a small knot on her navel (this seems to happen more than 80 to 90% of the time). We selected source points on the same channel and built a treatment from there.

The next week, Mary was walking without wobbling side to side and her eyes were brighter. When she started to speak, it was if a cloud had been lifted; the words came out smoothly without effort and they were articulate.

Herbal Treatment of Profections

The channel which is open during the year of the trauma has a corresponding organ. The year of trauma may be activated with herbal medicine by selecting an agent that enters the organ. This is then, combined with agents that move blood, calm the heart and open consciousness.

Profection in Summary

I combined the angle on the umbilicus that connected to the year of the trauma. I then connected it with the current hour and used the source points as expressions of the present. The idea: take an abstract representation of a time when a trauma occurred and mix it with the present, allowing them to collapse into each other, mixing and stirring the neurotransmitters that are connected to the experiences.

Time, space, and state remain an essential triangular component of the unfolding Dao. As it emerges from the one into two, reflecting back to include three, the ultimate potential remains. Once the three unfolds into the 1,000 things, the universe comes into being. Such methods that weave time, space, and state permit a return to source. As a threefold aspect of being transcendent, they have a reflection in the creation as heaven, humans, and earth—and— *spirit, vitality,* and *essence.*

DIVERGENT CHANNELS

The Language of Companionship is a unique one.
To reach someone through the Heart
is other than reaching them through words.
Besides words, allusions and arguments
the heart knows a hundred thousand ways to speak.
—Rumi

Divergent Channel Pathways

D ivergent channels course from the interior to the exterior, above and below, ever leaving and returning. The communication along these channels opens and closes self to the other, but also wards off pathogens, binding them safely, whether biological or psychological. Joining the source with the exterior, these channels link our essential self with the external world through the vehicles of nutritive, protective, and source qi.

Protective qi flows throughout the superficial interstices, connective tissues, and muscle structures during the daytime and the conscious waking periods. At night and during dreamtime, the protective qi flows inwardly throughout the deeper connective tissues and structures. Spreading out over the surface of the organs and throughout the deeper interstices, it connects to the deeply subjective states and the essence. When it flows on the surface, there are links to the objective world and the boundary between self and other. At the interior, it connects to the internal boundaries and conflicts.

As the protective qi moves to the interior during the night, through the dreamtime it brings resolution to many conflicts of the borderlands where we draw the lines of our existence. The nutritive vitality travels with the blood inside the vessels. This aspect of blood is constructive, traveling through the primary channels to provide nourishment. It provides a deep foundation typically undisturbed by external events. This tranquil, pure vitality moves through the channels on a diurnal basis in the same tempo whereby the sun moves through the sky. We follow the course of day and night, activity and rest, seeking connections that nourish others and ourselves, and which impresses meaning upon our lives. The sum of one's inherited and acquired source vitality rests deeply.

Deriving from one's parents, inherited vitality brings about conception. Such essence resembles *pneuma* more than fluid. This dynamic and rarified form of essence can be described as essence transformed into vitality with roots in the kidneys, and finding nuance within expression as *yin* and *yang*. Thus, the source vitality is the foundation of *yin* and *yang* within the human being. Source vitality like essence, requires nourishment through cultivation and protection by lifestyle. Exercise such as yoga and qi gung are efficient means of protecting, sustaining, and nourishing the source vitality.

Divergent channel pathways depart the surface and travel deep through the organs ultimately arriving at the crown of the head in the Thousand Meeting point, Du 20 (*bǎi huì* 百会). This pathway joins the paired *yin* and *yang* channels with their organs, the heart, the diaphragm, and the brain. Connecting our internal and external worlds, in the depths we find the patterns of self. At the surface, we find the patterns of connection with the environment. The protective vitality travels on the surface, the nutrient vitality flows in the channels, and the source vitality flows in the depths. Chapter 11 of the *Ling Shu* discusses the trajectory of the divergent channels, "An astute physician inspects carefully the condition of the channels … where the principle channel does not go, the divergent channel must go."

Three primary criteria for selecting divergent channel treatments include: 1) organic lesions, 2) chronic intermittent symptoms, and 3) psychosocial disorders. Once the appropriateness of a divergent channel treatment has been determined, the channel is selected based upon the site of pathology. For instance, for a stomach ulcer, use the stomach or spleen divergent channel. For psychosocial disorders, identify the primary organ and use its divergent channel or that of a related channel. Regarding chronic intermittent symptoms, consider arthritis, colitis, chronic fatigue syndrome, multiple sclerosis, and fibromyalgia. The pulse may be used for selecting a divergent channel. I often use the 6-channel method of Wang Shu-he (Morris 2003).

The Van Nghi school maintains that all divergent channels pass through the heart. We will use this point of view since divergent channels have powerful effects on the heart and mind. Further, I maintain that all divergents pass through the diaphragm, making it one of the prime pulse indicators for the use of a divergent channel treatment.

Divergent channels are wide ranging in application given the connection between the interior and the exterior. They provide systems whereby conflicts between the internal and external world are processed and transformed. The internal flow of vitality follows the trajectory of the *yin* channels—confluences one, two, and three travel upward, confluences four, five, and six flow downward. Since the Spiritual Axis does not discuss specific points, palpation can be used to determine which points are appropriate.

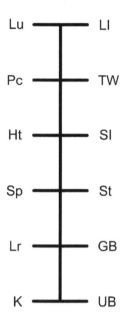

Figure 9: Channel Divergent Hierarchy

Reversals of the flow vitality, in terms of bodily and psychic functions, may be described as afflux and efflux. Afflux refers to a return or a flowing toward the head. Efflux is flowing toward the feet. Vitality moves as a form of information along the divergent channels from the exterior to the interior. As for effect, this movement takes place from the interior to the exterior, where the individual effects change upon the environs. The afflux type of reversal may involve affections such as oppression, anxiety, irritability, or sudden pain. Blushing and redness of the face due to anger, fear, or spicy food and alcohol are described in the *Su Wen* Ling Shu by the words *jue* afflux and *jueni* efflux or counterflow. Other conditions due to counterflow include bi syndromes and malignant or benign tumors (concretions and conglomerations).

In the *yin* channels, afflux moves with the channels as an upward movement, while efflux moves against the channels as downward. In the *yang* channels it is the reverse. The efflux moves with the channels, downward and outward. The afflux moves against the channels, upward and inward. The *yin* channels are the affective domain; they are in reversal when effective and objective criteria are used to control and dominate the affective experience. Whereas the *yang* channels are effective, imbued with the intent to reach out and make a difference.

In terms of the humors, cold afflux patients have cold feet or hands, they may also be hot, this is then called efflux since the heat is congesting the exterior. In either case, the six divergent channels are likely disturbed. Essentially, temperature disturbances at the extremities point towards some form of reversal in terms of afflux towards the interior or efflux towards the exterior.

We humans are the children of heaven and earth. As these children, we cannot avoid being influenced by nature. When spring and summer come, it changes and heat begins. When winter and autumn come, what dominates is cold from the environment. Psychologically, the afflux internalizes in the emotional realm. Efflux refers to the observation of events or "objects" occurring in the external world. Congestion and stagnation in these channels may occur when objective and subjective phenomena are unresolved.

This connection between the source vitality and the external objective events can be treated via the divergent channels because they connect the objective and the subjective, the affective and the effective, the internal and the external. They are the place where the ambiguity between the disparate poles of reality can be resolved physiologically, psychologically, and spiritually.

Divergent Channel Relationship to Nutritive and Protective

Divergent channels provide a means of communication between *yin* and *yang*. Nutritive travels inside the channel and protective travels outside the channels. Nutritive vitality relates with blood, while protective vitality has greater affinity with the general vitality. Further, nutritive vitality is *yin* and protective vitality is *yang*. Healthy communication between the surface and the interior, nutritive and protective vitality, general vitality and blood, all require that *yin* and *yang* be in harmonious communication.

This type of communication takes place between self and other, but also the interior and exterior of one's life. In a sense, we are speaking of the boundaries between self and other. It is these boundaries by which we define ourselves in the context of the social systems in which we evolve. When frustrations and stagnations happen within these zones, the divergent channels are active.

Features of Certain Divergent Channels

The hand triple warmer and the hand pericardium are the only divergent channels that travel downward. They are the channels related to ministerial fire. It is possible that divergent of the ministerial fire subdue the passions, leading it back to source. Such a strategy is important when the passions are overflowing, but also when there are too many interests in life.

Pulse Diagnosis of the Divergent Channels

Divergent channel pulses show poor communication between the interior and exterior. When pressing vertically, the pulse will be either deep or without root, that is, the pulse cannot be felt in the depth. The pulse may also be congested distally, in the middle or proximally. That is, when exploring along the length of the vessel, there is accumulation in a given area, it suggests that the qi is not moving upward or downward freely. This is a positive indicator for a divergent channel treatment. Such shapes may be described using terms for the eight extraordinary vessels. These include the *dai mai*, *yin qiao*, and *yang qiao* shapes. Other pulse shapes include the diaphragm, superficial palmar artery, and spillage pulses, which are felt on the palmar surface (Morris and Li 2010). The *yin wei* and *yang wei* pulse shapes also suggest poor communication between the interior and the exterior (Morris 2002). Lastly, pulses that are very close to the tendon flexor carpi radialis, or extended laterally upon the radial bone, suggest poor communication between the interior and the exterior. These can include the Six Channel pulses of Wang Shu-he, when located in a single position (Morris 2003).

Once the nature of the poor communication between the upper and lower or interior and exterior are established, then the selection of the channel may be considered. The six-channel pulse method may also be used here (Morris 2003). The carotid-radial ration is an excellent tool since it directly shows the distribution of qi and blood above and below, left and right. Also, palpation of the channels in general, or the rest of the sign-symptom complex, will guide the decision.

The function of the divergent channels, and their corresponding organs, serves to guide the clinical gaze. Consider, for instance, gastrointestinal dysfunction as a guide to the stomach divergent channel. Check the stomach pulse in the right middle position. Look for signals of divergent channel problems, such as the positive diaphragm or, most typically, a lack of root in the stomach position. Organic lesions can be typified by a slippery quality at the organ depth in the corresponding body area. The corresponding emotional factors may be addressed by using divergent channel treatments. The emotional component includes the effect of the pathway through the heart, diaphragm, and ultimately passing through the curious organ, the brain. If the pulse is very deep or superficial, then *luo* channel treatments may be useful in combination with the channel divergents. In this case, the lack of communication between the interior and exterior through the divergent pathways may be indicated by pulse qualities such as empty, floating-yielding, deep, and changing amplitude.

Diaphragm Pulse

The diaphragm pulse bulges between the middle and upper burners. Palpate it by placing the index finger in the area between the distal (*cùn*) and middle (*guān*) positions (see Figure 10), or, roll into the diaphragm area from the middle and distal positions (Hammer 2001). When the diaphragm area has a tense and full quality, it suggests suppressed emotions. Divergent channels traverse the diaphragm, and they are useful for quickly opening the diaphragm. Aside from suppressed emotions, latent pathogens can easily be bound into the region above the diaphragm which is called the membrane-source, which also refers to a pleurodiaphragmatic interspace (*mó yuán* 膜原) (Wen and Seifert 2000).

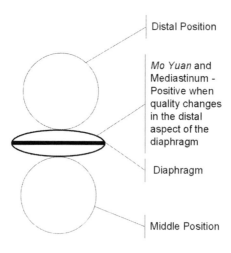

Figure 10: Diaphragm and Mo Yuan

This image shows the diaphragm pulse with its subset, the *mó yuán* 膜原, which is palpated by placing the index finger upon the apex of the diaphragm pulse and rolling distally. There must be a change in quality for it to be positive. The treatment is then based upon the nature of those qualities. The reason for this is that the *mó yuán* 膜原 qualities are usually latent or hidden and often do not present in the framework of the whole picture.

Spillage Pulse (*yì mài* 溢脉)

The arrival of all divergent pathways at DU 20 *(bǎi huì* 百会) is represented in an area just beyond the distal (*cùn*) position, on the thenar eminence of the thumb. It is a subset of the long pulse that appears in a notch on the thenar eminence of the thumb. Passing over its original position *cùn*, when it is only long in the upper area, it is called "spillage pulse" (*yì mài* 溢脉) (Morris and Li 2010). Because the pulse extends beyond its normal range, it is suggestive of poor communication between the upper and the lower, the exterior and the interior. Hammer (2001) places his "neuropsychological" pulse in this region. However, he locates the neuropsychological pulse solely in the notch upon the thenar eminence of the thumb. The spillage pulse easily covers more terrain, as a pulse extending onto the fleshy portion of the thenar eminence may present differently. Hammer interprets the "neuropsychological" pulse similarly to the "spillage pulse" (*yì mài* 溢脉) of Li Shi-zhen, in terms of psychological state.

A spillage pulse on one wrist seems to be an ipsilateral indicator of heightened sensitivity for various points around the cranium. Points that I find to be most sensitive tend to be along the gallbladder channel, then the *san jiao*, and least often is the *du* channels in the region of the cranium. The spillage pulse corrects, and is no longer apparent, most consistently with the gallbladder channel. Cranial and neck point tenderness can be used to confirm divergent involvement. This is because of the congestion due to the lack of free flow from the upper to the lower.

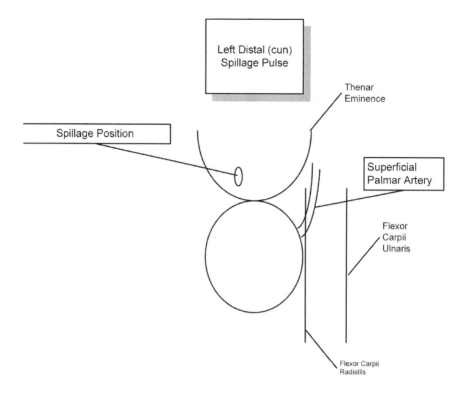

Figure 11: Spillage Pulse

As a curious organ, the brain has affinity with marrow and essence. The GB is the vehicle by which influences from the exterior may finally penetrate the essence. This is made apparent by the function of GB 39 (*xuán zhōng* 悬钟), the influential point for marrow.

Example: If the left spillage pulse is present, palpate the channels of the gallbladder, *san jiao*, urinary bladder, and *du* throughout the cranium. Use the corresponding Divergent channel *he*-sea point for the area of predominant tenderness. *i.e.,* the GB. Palpate GB 34 (*yáng líng quán* 阳陵泉) for tenderness and check both cranial tender points and the spillage pulse. The tenderness along the channel pathway and the pulse should both diminish.

Placement of the Vessel

The pulse is a three-dimensional field. Communication between the surface and the interior can be suggested by depth, placement radius to ulna, and distribution distal to proximal. The course vibrations at the organ depth suggest damage to organ tissue. If the pulse is very deep or superficial, then the use of *Luo* channels in conjunction with divergents is often a useful intervention.

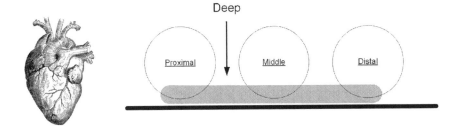

Figure 12: Deep Pulse

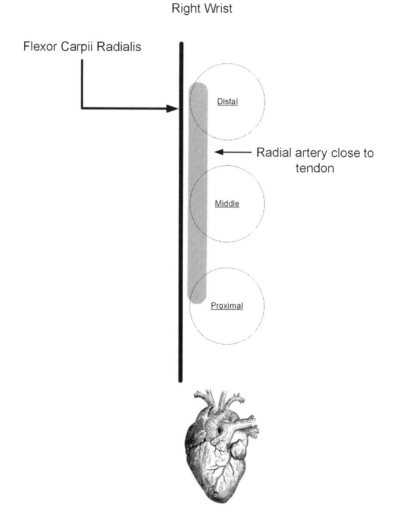

Figure 13: Artery Close to Tendon

Divergent Channel Pulse Sequence

The movement of the divergent channels from I-VI is from posterior to anterior in the leg channels and posterior to anterior in
the arm channels. The movement is from exterior to interior and
returning to the surface of *yin* in the *tai yin* aspect of metal.

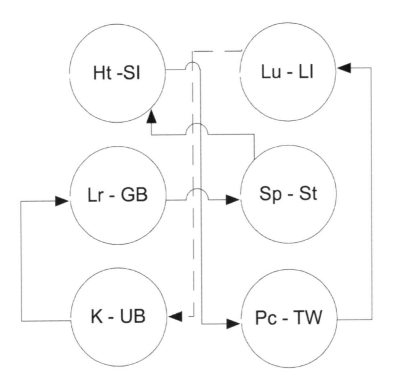

Figure 14: Sequence of Divergent Pulses

The sequence of the divergent channels mapped onto the pulse demonstrates a connection between the left and right sides. Consider the divergent channels when there is a disparity between the pulses side to side.

Consider also that the divergent channels carry essential substances from the lower burner upward. While this may be a useful exercise, the pulses that show the movement of essential substances above and below, inside and out, are the bell-weather for divergent channel applications. After that, the normal pulses of the organs are useful for selecting the appropriate channel. The overall emotion and location of lesion at the interior are key for selecting the divergent channel. Lastly, the Six Channel method, as I have built it, from Wang Shu-he's *Pulse Classic*, is useful (Morris 2003).

Applying the five transformations, the small death return from metal to water recapitulates mystery traditions throughout the world.

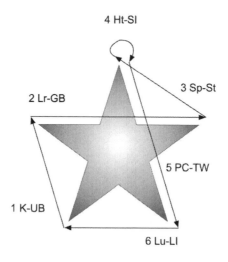

Figure 15: Sequence of Divergent Channels

The divergent channels applied to the five transformations are more chaotic in their presentation than when they are applied to the surface anatomy arrangement of the 12 channels. In the latter, the divergent channels progress from posterior to anterior beginning with the leg and then the arm. The first circuit is the water channels of the Kidney and Urinary Bladder. The second circuit includes the wood channels of the liver and gall bladder. The third circuit is the anterior earth pair of the spleen and stomach. The fourth circuit begins in the posterior aspect of the heart and small intestine, then moves to the anterior, the *san jiao* and pericardium pair, and lastly, the lung and large intestine channels.

Acupuncture Treatment of the Divergent Channels

The pure heart of acupuncture is transmitted through the Yellow Emperor's Canon, which states, "The poor physician considers the study of the channels easy, the advanced physician considers it difficult." Humans are born, live, have disease, and die via the channel pathways. They are the beginning and end of this medicine.

Psyche may somatize into any tissue, and since the divergent channels are a place where the communication between the interior and the exterior takes place—the self and the other, they serve as a repository for deeply held traumatic history. Thus, caution should be used with divergent channel treatments. Connecting the superficies and the depths, they can stir up material that is difficult for the patient to work through.

The divergent channels are a location where psychosocial and connective tissue armoring can allow for avoidance or compensation, which can lead to a binding of vitality. When these channels are treated, the person may decompensate and a regression in the case can easily take place. The question will be whether it is on the road to improvement or a worsening of the condition. For these reasons, it is important to become familiar with the patient prior to using divergent channels.

Point locations on the divergent channels vary depending upon source. Two methods of point selection for the divergent pathways tend to be in use. One uses the departure from the *he*-sea points, the other uses departure in the large joints of the torso. The divergent channels reconvene in the head and neck area. Van Nghi has interpreted the "window of the sky" points as the upper reunion points of the channel divergents. It makes most sense to palpate the pathway of the divergent to identify the areas where the vitality is stagnating or entangled. One method of divergent channel treatment is to use the *he*-sea points (at the elbows and knees) in combination with the window of the sky points around the head, neck, and shoulders. The lower meeting points may be constructed from the *he*-sea points or major points at the hips and shoulders. The upper meeting points may be constructed from the window of the sky points or *yang* channel points in the head.

Wilhelm Reich, a student of Sigmund Freud, conceived of the character and trauma of life to bind into the tissues—a view that was in stark contrast to the archetypal focus of the Jungian perspective. Character armoring involves attitudes used to block against emotional excitations. This generates corresponding muscle rigidity and interferes with emotional contact (Reich 1980a). The application of this concept by Reich led him to combining breathing techniques with various methods to stress the tissue sites where the armoring could be observed. This might occur through holding postures for extended periods of time in order to get tissues to release, or it might be deep tissue work similar to Rolfing in order to get a discharge. The discharge often involved shaking or a state called "vibratory." The important activity when discharge is occurring is breathing and for the practitioner to observe where the muscle structures are becoming tense, so that the patient may be directed to release those structures so that a whole vibratory state may unfold.

Confluence	Channel - Organs	Lower Reunion			
		French	Japanese	R. Low	Yitian Ni
Water 1	UB - K	UB 40 - K 10	UB 40 - K 10	UB 54	UB 40 - K10
Wood 2	GB - Lr	GB 30 - Liv 12	GB 34 - Liv 8	Lr 2	Gb 30 - Lr 3
Earth 3	St - Sp	St 30 - Sp 12	St 36 - Ht 1	St 30	St 30 - Sp 12
Imperial Fire 4	SI - Ht	SI 10 - Ht 1	SI 8 - Ht 1	GB 22	SI 10 - Ht 1
Minestrial Fire 5	SJ - PC	SJ 16 - P 1	TB 10 - P 3	-	Du 20 - GB 22
Metal 6	LI - Lu	LI 15 - Lu1	LI 11 - Lu 5	St 12	- / Lu 1

Confluence	Channel - Organs	Upper Reunion			
		French	Japanese	R. Low	Yitian NI
Water 1	UB - K	UB 10	UB 1 - UB 11	UB 10	UB 10
Wood 2	GB - LR	GB 20 - GB 9	GB 1	GB 1	GB 1
Earth 3	ST - SP	UB 1 - ST 1	ST 1	UB 1	UB 1
Imperial Fire 4	SI - HT	UB 1	UB 1	UB 1	UB 1
Minestrial Fire 5	SJ - PC	DU 20	GB 12	SJ 16	-
Metal 6	LI - LU	LI 18	ST 12	LI 18	LI 18

Table 6: Divergent Point Considerations from Various Traditions

Window of the Sky			
Tai Yang	UB 10	SI 16	Expressive
Shao Yang	SJ 17	SJ 16	Hesitant
Yang Ming	ST 9	LI 18	Inactive

Doorway to the Earth		
Tai Yin	SP 12	REN 1
Shao Yin	K 11	REN 2
Jue Yin	LR 12	REN 4
Tai Yang	UB 40	UB 35
Shao Yang	GB 30	DU 4
Yang Ming	ST 30	

Table 7: Additional Point Possibilities for Channel

The reason for the discrepancies among these schools is because the Ling Shu did not specify many of the points. It specified UB 40—so that is the same in both systems.

Once points on the divergent channel are placed, the pulse can be assessed for the eight extraordinary vessels that arise as the body attempts to compensate for the materials arising during the divergent channel treatment. The use of the eight extraordinary vessels, in conjunction with treatments that dredge the channels, is critical in my opinion. When we dredge these channels, they are not solely vehicles for material substances. Rather, they also lodge pathogens, both internal and external. Thus, I surmise that historical material, biological as well as psychosocial, lodge in the channels, especially the divergent channels.

All treatment that contacts a deep wound has potential for acting beyond the capacity of the patient. A high level of sensitivity is essential. Along with a high awareness within the clinical interaction as to the capacity and willingness of the patient to pursue treatment with the practitioner, there is a need for the practitioner to be able to assess whether the treatment is producing desired results or not, especially in the context of and aggravation. The great homeopath Constantine Herring provides significant assistance in the effort to understand whether a patient who has a mild aggravation is on the path towards wellness or there is a medical error at play.

Herbal Treatment of the Divergent Channels

This method requires using agents which move upward such as aerial plant parts and diaphoretics. These are then combined with medicinals that have a down-bearing function such as carminatives and diuretics. There are many agents that open the diaphragm in the carminative class. Dr. Shen's favorite herb to open the diaphragm, and in my opinion, free the divergent channels is sweet gum, Fructus Liquidambaris sp. (*lù lù tong* 路路通).

HERRING'S LAW OF CURE

The likelihood of an abreaction to treatment is ever present. Given such circumstance, it becomes necessary, therefore, to have tools for the purpose of understanding whether a case is improving or not.

Given an uncomfortable response to treatment, how do we know whether the condition is better or worse? If the luminosity in the eyes (spirit) improves, it suggests the case is going in the right direction. If there is a dulling of spirit, more caution is required. If a patient calls with a concern about a reaction to treatment, it is necessary to determine whether it is indeed that treatment which caused the problem. Inquiry into the patient's behaviors and diet at the time of the reaction is necessary. There are other tools for understanding the direction and progression of a patient's condition.

Homeopathy has a relatively well-developed model for assessing aggravations, and whether they represent an improvement or a worsening of the condition. Herring's law of cure states that curing takes place from:

- the top down,
- the present to the past,
- the interior to the exterior,
- and the most important organ to the least important organ.

Not in a particular order, any one of these vectors may be analyzed to determine whether an aggravation is resulting in improvement or a worsening of the condition.

If the center of pathology moves toward more important organs or toward the center, the condition may be worsening. Tongue and pulse findings help this inquiry. For instance, if the pulses were uneven before the treatment, and then became more smooth and moderate, it suggests improvement. If the tongue were shiny and developed a thin coat, this might be considered an improvement. The reverse would portend a downturn in the case.

Time frames are to be considered. Let's say the next day after treatment the patient feels a downturn, possibly sleeping for hours. But on the following day, the patient feels spectacular. Upon return to the clinic, I observe greater clarity of spirit in the patient's eyes. This was a beneficial form of healing crisis.

In summary, healing moves from the inside to the outside, top to bottom, most important organ to least important organ, and from the most recent to the most past. The divergent channels are an appropriate mode of address for the healing processes described by Herring, as they follow the trajectory of disease and health he describes.

SUMMARY

This book is an attempt to describe a way of connecting between self and the world in which that self moves. The imprints taking place throughout the course of life are significant to the extent meaning is assigned to them by the native.

We have explored variations upon self and the treatment of the well patient. Such an approach requires the mere connection and speaking to that which is present in the person as an awareness of being. My two favorite approaches are the five element (which I translate as transformation) approaches, as practiced by Worsley, along with the three treasures herbal model.

Three tools for approaching traumatic experiences have been addressed. The eight extraordinary vessels are useful additions to any other method, as they enhance the adaptive capacities. The profection is presented here for the first time. It is a historical east-west integration whereby chronotopes are explored for the purpose of connecting to, and allowing transformation of, traumatic and other significant life events. The third is a framework for considered application of the divergent channels and pulses that can inform such thought.

Successful treatment can be viewed on the basis of clinical outcomes, the achievement of therapeutic goals, and the evidence of effective treatment. The nature of self-realization, becomes a rather ephemeral feature of the clinical relationship in the practice of Chinese medicine. As the connection to self develops, more possibilities are created toward wellness throughout the range of life experiences. The degree to which we are connected to self is the degree to which we connect to the other, in a fundamental loving way.

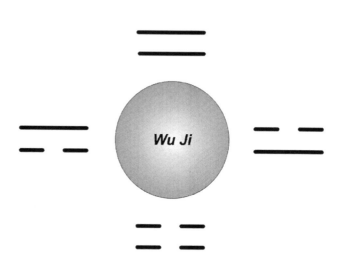

BIBLIOGRAPHY

Anderson, Walter Truett. 1997. *The Future of the Self: Inventing the Postmodern Person.* New York: Jeremy P. Tarcher/Putnam.

Bergson, Henri Louis. 1960. *Time and Free Will.* New York: Harper & Brothers.

Combs, Allan. 2002. *The Radiance of Being: Understanding the Grand Integral Vision; Living the Integral Life.* St Paul, MN: Paragon House.

Fodor, Nandor. 1949. *The Search For the Beloved. A Clinical Investigation of the Trauma of Birth and Pre-Natal Conditioning.* New Hyde Park, NY: University Books.

Foucault, Michel. 1963. *The Birth of the Clinic an Archeology of Medical Perception.* Translated by Sheridan Smith. New York: Vintage.

Fraser, J.T. 1986. "The Problems of Exporting Faust," in *Time, Science, and Society in China and the West: (The Study of Time V).* Edited by J.T. Fraser, N. Lawrence and F.C. Haber. Amherst: University of Massachusetts Press.

Gilligan, Carol. 1993. *In a Different Voice: Psychological Theory and Women's Development.* Cambridge: Harvard University Press.

Goffman, Erving. 1959. *The Presentation of Self in Everyday Life.* Garden City, New York: Doubleday.

Grof, Stanislav. 1985. *Beyond the Brain (Birth, Death and Transcendence in Psychotherapy).* Albany: State University of New York.

Grof, Stanislav. 1993. *The Holotropic Mind: The Three Levels of Human Consciousness and How They Shape Our Lives.* San Francisco: Harper.

Grof, Stanislav. 1975. *Realms of the Human Unconscious: Observations from LSD Research.* New York: Viking Press.

Hammer, Leon. 2001. *Chinese Pulse Diagnosis, A Contemporary Approach.* Seattle: Eastland Press.

Janov, Arthur. 1970. *The Primal Scream.* New York: Dell Publishing.

Jarrett, Lonnie. 1990. *Nourishing Destiny: The Inner Tradition of Chinese Medicine.* Spirit Path Press.

Keeney, Bradford. 2011. "Why Therapy is Jazz," in *Circulus: Journal for Creative Transformation.* Vol. 1 (1).

Kohlberg, L. 1981. *Essays on Moral Development.* San Francisco: Harper & Row.

Lake, F. 1978. "Birth Trauma, Claustrophobia and LSD Therapy," in *The Undivided Self:* 10-29.

Li, Shizhen. 2008. *The Qi Jing Ba Mai Kao (Studies on the Eight Extraordinary Vessels).* Chinese Medicine Database 2006 [cited April 20 2008].

http://db.cm-db.com/translation/view/6.

Lowen, Alexander. 1972. *Depression and the Body: The Biological Basis of Faith and Reality.* New York: Coward, McCann & Geoghegan.

Morris, William. 2002. "Eight Extra Vessel Pulse Diagnosis: A Path to Effective Treatment," in *Acupuncture Today.* Vol. 03 (1).

Ming, L. I. (1988). Inner Teachings of Taoism. Boulder, CO, Shambhala Publications

Morris, William. 2003. "Neoclassical Pulse Diagnosis and the Six Channels," in *Acupuncture Today.* Vol. 4 (4).

Morris, William and Shen-qing, Li. 2010. *Li Shi Zhen's Pulse Studies: An Illustrated Guide*. Edited by Mark Mandot. Beijing: People's Medical Publishing House.

Painter, Jack. 1987. *Technical Manual of Deep Wholistic Bodywork: Postural Integration*. Mill Valley: Jack Painter.

Piaget, Jean. 1960. *The Child's Conception of the World*. Translated by Joan Tomlinson and Andrew Tomlinson. Patterson, NJ: Littlefield, Adams.

Rank, Otto. 1993. *The Trauma of Birth*. Reprint of Kegan Paul 1933 edition. New York: Dover.

Reich, Wilhelm. 1980a. *Character Analysis*. Translated by Vincent Carfagno. 3rd Edition. New York: Farrar, Straus and Giroux.

Reich, Wilhelm. 1980b. *The Mass Psychology of Fascism*. Translated by Vincent Carfagno. 3rd Edition. New York: Farrar, Straus and Giroux.

Rogers, Carl. 1961. *On Becoming a Person*. New York: Houghton Mifflin.

Rolf, Ida. 1989. *Rolfing: Reestablishing the Natural Alignment and Structural Integration of the Human Body for Vitality and Well-Being*. Rochester VT: Healing Arts Press.

Sydenham, Thomas. 1979. *The Works of Thomas Sydenham, M.D.* Reprint of the 1848 and 1850 London Sydenham Society volumes 1 and 2 edition. Birmingham Alabama: Classics of Medicine Library.

Tulku, Tarthang. 1984. *Love of knowledge*. Berkeley, CA: Dharma Press.

Unschuld, Paul. 1986. *Nan-Ching: The Classic of Difficult Issues*. Translated by Paul Unschuld, Medicine in China. Berkeley, CA University of California Press. (Original edition, 200 C.E.).

Valens, Vettius. 2004. *Vettius Valens: The Anthology Book IV* (*c.* 160 CE). Translated by Robert Schmidt. Edited by Robert Schmidt. Vol. Volume XI, Greek Track Columbia, MD: Project Hindsight.

Wade, Jenny. 1996. *Change of Mind: A Holonomic Theory of the Evolution of Consciousness.* Albany: State University of New York.

Wang, Bing. 1997. *Yellow Emperor's Canon of Internal Medicine.* Translated and edited by Andrew Qi Wu and Nelson Liansheng Wu. Beijing: China Science and Technology Press.

Wen, Jian Min, and Garry Seifert. 2000. *Warm Disease Theory (Wen Bing Xue).* Brookline, MA: Paradigm Publications.

Wilson, Robert Anton. 1987. *Wilhelm Reich in Hell: Knowledge of Tomorrow.* Tempe, AZ: New Falcon.

Worsley, J. R. 1990. *Traditional Acupuncture: Volume 2, Traditional Diagnosis.* United Kingdom: The College of Traditional Acupuncture.

Yang, Joseph Changqing, and William Morris. 2007. "Shen Harmony: The normal mental condition in Chinese Medicine." *Acupuncture Today*, Vol. 9 (10).

Made in the USA
San Bernardino, CA
10 November 2015